COMPLETE CHAKRAS FOR BEGINNERS

The Solution to Chakras Healing and Balancing Your Body, Mind, and Positive Energies

By

Tracey Germon

Table of Contents

FOREWARD

This is a great book if you're just starting to get to know or just want to work with your chakras. Refreshingly, it discusses the full twelve chakra system unlike most books on this topic that usually just cover the seven main chakra points. It's important beginners understand there are energy centers beyond the body and how they are best used to improve spiritual wellbeing. There are many different ways to heal or maintain the balance of your chakra system, and a lot of these are provided in this book.

I found Complete Chakras for Beginners easy to follow, while providing lots of information allowing the reader to easily connect the dots, also giving plenty of tips and examples for the reader to try out. A great little book for anybody new to learning the chakras or just wanting a refresher. A must have in your library of spiritual development.

I have known Tracey now for many years and in that time, we always found ourselves discussing healing systems and the effect on the physical, spiritual and emotional body. Tracey, as a healer, loves to delve deeply into all these areas to better enhance her own life and others for wellbeing on all levels. It comes as no surprise to me that she finally has put together her wisdom in this book on the chakras. As a T.V. and Radio International psychic medium and healer myself of over 15 years, it's really exciting and refreshing to have something simply and informatively put together when so many people now are opening up their spirituality to better understand themselves, other than just the physical aspects of themselves.

Anne Scholes

International Psychic Medium,

TV and Radio personality, Angelic Reiki and Reiki Healer

Owner of Annegelic Bliss Holistic and Wellness Centre

INTRODUCTION

Congratulations on purchasing *Complete Chakras for Beginners: The Solution to Chakras Healing and Balancing Your Body, Mind, and Positive Energies,* and thank you for doing so.

The following chapters will discuss everything you will ever need to know about your chakras. You will learn how to know when your chakras are unhealthy or unbalanced and how to rebalance your chakras and make them healthy again.

Your chakras are centers of energy responsible for providing energy and balance for your body. There are different chakras for each area of your body, and all of them work together to keep you healthy and balanced. If even one chakra is not performing efficiently at the correct rate for that chakra, the entire body will be thrown off balance. Your chakras all work together inside of you to keep your energies flowing freely, and every chakra depends on every other chakra to fulfill its role in keeping the energy systems of your body healthy and flowing well.

You will learn how to determine when one or more of your chakras is unbalanced or unhealthy. An unbalanced chakra can be underperforming or overperforming, and either of these can upset your natural balance. You will also learn various ways you can heal your chakras, one at a time or all together, and the best ways to keep your chakras balanced and healthy. When you have achieved this, you will be able to live a happy, productive life, free of the problems you feel when your chakras need attention.

There are plenty of books on this subject on the market, so thanks again for choosing this one! Every effort was made to ensure it is full of as much useful information as possible, and please enjoy!

1

CHAPTER:
Introduction to The Chakras

The word 'chakra' has been with us since ancient times. The word translates literally to 'spinning disk.' Your chakras are centers of energy inside your body, spinning wheels of energy responsible for providing energy to various parts of your body in order to energize the body as a whole. Chakras are found inside your body as places where channels or meridians meet and cross.

Long before modern times, the system of chakras was well known in ancient Indian practices. The ancient healers verbally passed down the knowledge they had of the chakras as part of the tradition of Eastern philosophy. The Hindu religion used the concept of the chakra in its ritual and spiritual traditions. In their traditions, the chakra was anything with a cyclical or circular motion or aspect to itself. The wheel of time, the wheel of life, and the wheel of creation are all cyclical naturally. In their religious traditions, the highest God was depicted as a wheel because he is the natural source of the order and regularity of the rhythm of life.

Chakras and chakra healing regained popularity in the mid-to - late twentieth century as part of the New Age revival seeking more natural, holistic healing as a way of life. The followers wanted a pure and traditional way of living. Their way of living used the function of each of the chakras in an association with various physical functions in the body, the aspect of consciousness, classical elements, and other characteristics distinguishing one chakra from another. These are the ideas the ancient healers of India used so many centuries ago.

As the New Age followers taught us, and as the ancient healers knew centuries ago, each chakra has a power providing energy and vitality to one particular area of the human body. They also provide energy for the physical, mental, and emotional movement and function of your body. The movement brought a renewed interest in the study of chakras and how they affect our everyday lives. The followers of the New Age movement were looking for a life free from the chemicals and medications people were using to make their minds and bodies feel better and hopefully heal from diseases and ailments. Instead, they sought the ancient, natural ways of keeping the mind and body healthy by trying to avoid diseases and illnesses. The basic belief they borrowed from the ancient healers of the East was that energy was released during the creation of the world, an energy force known as the Kundalini. This force is present in all of us, lying dormant and sleeping at the base of the spine until it is awakened. When awoken, the energy will spread through all the chakras in the body until it reaches the top of the head, where it leaves the body and connects with the higher spiritual powers of the universe. This is how the aura is created, that imperceptible life force surrounding all people.

Sometimes your chakras may become out of balance or may close completely. They may also become too widely open or spin too slowly or quickly. This causes the energy to flow through them improperly, making it unable to flow up the spine and through the body in a manner that keeps the body and the mind functioning at its best levels. The force of life, the 'chi,' become non-productive and stagnates inside the body, and this will cause health-related issues. These issues will also affect your emotional and mental health. If a chakra is not healthy for whatever reason, it can lead to disease or illness in the area of the body governed by that chakra. When you heal and unblock the chakras, these issues can be resolved. When you make a conscious effort to unblock your chakras, you begin to take back control of your own mental, emotional, and physical health and well-being. Your health and well-being on all levels are directly affected by the health of your chakras. If the foods you eat are not the right kinds to nourish your body, you will not take in the correct energy to fuel your chakras. If you are feeling depressed, this will disturb the energy flow to the chakras. If you constantly suppress your emotions such as anger or keep your opinions to yourself instead of speaking your mind, you will block the flow of energy to the chakras. Even being angry too often or overly opinionated can hurt the performance of your chakras.

Your body will send out signals that a particular chakra is blocked and needs cleansing and balancing. If you have problems sleeping, have difficulty concentrating, lack motivation, or fail to accomplish your goals, then you most likely have a blocked chakra. Unhealthy chakras can also lead to poor social skills, an inability to express oneself, depression and isolation. You should not heal a chakra and then resume your former unhealthy lifestyle, and this is important to remember. The energy put into cleansing and unblocking your chakras is not a goal but a way of life. Once you put effort into cleansing the chakras and optimizing overall balance and health, that effort must be continued if this new way of life is to be maintained. Keeping the chakras healthy involves many things, such as the colors you wear and the foods you eat. Different forms of exercise will help keep your chakras balanced. Letting go of the past will bring you to a better level of energy in your life. Clearing out any clutter surrounding you, both mentally and physically, will also greatly improve the health of your chakras.

So, when you decide to heal your chakras, you decide to begin living a healthy life full of energy and balance. This new lifestyle will soon become second nature and will lead to a wonderful rebirth for you. As humans, we pick up so much negativity from the world around us that it is no wonder our bodies suffer. But with daily practice and continuous effort, your chakras will be healthy and balanced, and you will be on your way to enjoying life as it should be enjoyed.

2
CHAPTER:
The Twelve Chakras

In order to appreciate what they do for you, it is important you know and understand your twelve chakras. Having familiarity with the twelve chakras will greatly enhance your ability to heal and balance them. In the twelve-chakra system, five of the chakras are actually located outside of your body, and they are responsible for keeping you grounded to the earth while helping you receive energy from the universe. The other seven chakras are located in your body along your spinal column and up to the top of your head. Your lower chakras are physical, while the higher ones are spiritual. The Heart Chakra is the meeting point for the two theories in your body, and it aligns with both physical and spiritual aspects of the chakras.

All living beings are one small part of a large complete system. Imagine that running along your spine is a thin wire stretching through you all the way up into the heavens and all the way down to about three feet below the surface of the earth. This wire keeps you grounded and allows you to receive energy flow. With twelve chakras, you can draw on the powerful energies lying outside of your body. This will also enable you to be in touch with the entire array of dimensions making up the human experience. In many of the ancient traditions, the sky and earth energies were believed to be a natural part of the human body.

Each of the chakras is aligned with a particular color, and the colors follow the spectrum of colors found in the rainbow, adding in gold and platinum. For the highest chakras, a combination of colors is used, referred to as iridescence or opalescence. Each chakra has a name and particular characteristics. Each is aligned with a particular part of the body and controls the health of that part of the body. Your chakras will work together to balance your body. Energy flows in them and through them to each other. They process and contain all the energy flowing into and through your body. The color of the chakra is also found in the aura surrounding your body. The intensity of these colors is directly affected by your overall health. A healthy, vibrant person will have an aura glowing with bright, strong colors. The colors representing unhealthy chakras will fade due to illness, stress, anger, or sadness.

THE EARTH STAR CHAKRA – This is the first of the twelve chakras and is actually found below your feet, outside of your body, about two to three feet below ground. This chakra is a projection of your system of energy outside your body. It is also responsible for helping you gather energy from the earth, as it directly connects you to the earth. When this chakra and your connection to it are strong and healthy, you will feel well-grounded and substantial. When this chakra is weak or your connection to it is failing, you will feel off-balance, and your head might feel too light and airy. When you develop a stronger, deeper connection with this chakra, you will more easily pull energy through this chakra on the days you need an extra burst of energy. This chakra will help draw out negativity you have collected throughout the day. Your root chakra will be healthier. You will have a stronger connection to the earth, and a better awareness of nature and your surroundings. The Earth Star Chakra is best healed with the use of meditation. There is some difference of opinion on the color of the Earth Star Chakra, with choices ranging from black to brown to brick red. It is best for you to meditate and decide which color feels truer to you.

THE ROOT CHAKRA – The Root Chakra is found at the base of your spine and is the center of your security, your basic needs, and your survival. The element of the Root Chakra is earth. Its theme is 'to be.' The Root Chakra governs your feet, legs, and bowels. The Crown Chakra balances the

Root Chakra in your body. The color representing the Root Chakra is red, since it is a completely physical color. Red promotes feelings of connection to the earth and of being grounded, so it works along with the Earth Star Chakra, as the two work together to keep you grounded physically and spiritually. Red will make you feel vigilant, alert, and primal. This is the very foundation of the entire system of energy inside of your body. It is also the chakra storing all the excess energy for the other chakras. If your Root Chakra is blocked, closed, unhealthy, or spinning excessively, it will give off definite symptoms. The physical problems can include problems with the legs, feet, lower back, bladder, or colon. You will suffer from digestive issues such as irritable bowel syndrome. You will have weakness in your lower limbs, or you will feel ungrounded. You might be nervous, fearful, greedy, or possessive. You will harbor irrational fears about your own safety, and you will probably have financial problems.

THE SACRAL CHAKRA -- Your second chakra holds the key to your deepest emotions and sensations. It controls how you express yourself and how you hold your emotions within your body. This chakra also controls your potential creativity as well as the balance of dark and light inside of you. The Sacral Chakra is found deep within the lower part of your abdomen, under your belly button. The corresponding color is orange, and its element is water. The theme of the Sacral Chakra is 'to feel,' and it corresponds to the kidneys, bladder, hips, lower back, and the reproductive system. The Throat Chakra balances the Sacral Chakra. When the Sacral Chakra is unhealthy in any way, you will suffer illnesses of the kidneys, bladder, or the reproductive system. Your emotions will be unbalanced, and you will feel confusion or shame over sexual matters or other intimate issues with your body, including harboring guilty feelings over things you enjoy doing. You might also suffer from various addictions to make you feel better about yourself. Your Sacral Chakra is responsible for your sexuality and creativity. When your Sacral Chakra is healthy, you will feel passionate, friendly, and fulfilled. You will exude feelings of abundance, pleasure, joy, and wellness. When you feel free to express your personal creativity and love for your body, your Sacral Chakra will be healthy. A blocked Sacral Chakra will cause you to feel creatively uninspired or emotionally unstable. The Sacral Chakra is aligned with orange, because this is the color of creativity and energy. Orange gives people a sense of warmth and security, and it's associated with thoughts and feelings of passion, pleasure, and sexuality. Orange makes people feel abundant, sensual, and safe. You need to maintain personal equilibrium while allowing creativity, pleasures, and emotions to flow freely to keep your Sacral Chakra healthy. Your Sacral Chakra grows stronger when you encourage a deep emotional connection with other people and healthy, honest expression of yourself.

THE SOLAR PLEXUS CHAKRA – Inside the upper part of your abdomen, just under your belly button, is your Solar Plexus Chakra. Here is where your inner fire begins and grows to ignite your self-confidence and willpower. Yellow is associated with the Solar Plexus Chakra, and its theme is 'to do.' Its element is fire, and it aligns with your gallbladder, spleen, pancreas, liver, and your stomach. The Third Eye Chakra balances the Solar Plexus Chakra. If your Solar Plexus Chakra is unhealthy in any way you will experience problems controlling your emotions, and you may have no willpower. You will either have poor self-esteem or an exaggerated sense of your own self-importance. You will alternate between feeling angry and insecure. You will struggle with bloating, gas, indigestion, fatigue, and weight control issues. If you are overly confident, you might have a protruding midsection making it look like you are strutting when you walk. But if you suffer from a lack of self-confidence, you will stand and walk with rolled shoulders as you fold forward looking timid or defeated. The color yellow is strongly emotional. It gives you feelings of confidence and friendliness. Yellow will bring you thoughts and feelings of self-esteem, courage, and optimism. The color yellow will make you feel prepared, capable, and stimulated in the same way a healthy Solar Plexus Chakra will. This chakra rules your self-esteem, balance, and action, focusing on personal power, commitment, and individual willpower. It governs any issues with your stomach, your digestive system, and metabolism.

THE HEART CHAKRA – This chakra is centrally located in the center of your chest and is balanced by all the other chakras. Your Heart Chakra is the chakra controlling the way you express caring and love for all people. Green is the color for the Heart Chakra, and its element is air. Your Heart Chakra aligns with your circulatory system and your arms, lungs, and heart. The theme of this chakra is 'to love.' An unhealthy Heart Chakra will cause issues with your respiratory system, circulatory system, and heart disease. You will often feel lonely, co-dependent, jealous, and sad. You will sacrifice your own desires to take care of other people. You might also hold grudges against others. Your Heart Chakra lies in the actual and metaphysical heart of your body and is the center of the seven internal chakras. This chakra needs unconditional love to function properly at all times. When your life is full of discord, when you have been betrayed by another, when you feel unrequited love for another, or when grief is crushing you, your Heart Chakra will be unbalanced and unhealthy. The color green will give you feelings of good health and well-being. It fuels thoughts and feelings of compassion, kindness, and love, and will make you feel healthy, alert, and empathetic. Your physical-self and your spiritual-self come together in the Heart Chakra. This is where you will feel spiritual awareness, forgiveness, compassion, and love.

THE THROAT CHAKRA -- Your own personal truths are honored and expressed in the Throat Chakra. Located in the throat, the Sacral Chakra is its balancing chakra. Its corresponding color is blue, and its element is ether. Your Throat Chakra aligns with your mouth, jaw, thyroid, shoulders, neck, and throat. Its theme is 'to speak.' If your Throat Chakra is unhealthy in any way you might feel pain or tightness in your jaw, shoulders, or throat. Your thyroid gland may be diseased. You will either talk constantly or suffer through long periods of silence. You might find it difficult to speak the truth and that lying is so much easier. You may have problems speaking to other people or communicating your real thoughts and feelings. Your Throat Chakra is particularly delicate and excessively hearing other people tell you your opinions are wrong or do not matter can cause damage to this chakra. If your personal expression is suppressed it can cause you to hide deep within yourself or to close off all expression. Your Throat Chakra prefers open communication expressed with encouragement in a safe environment. The Throat Chakra promotes feelings of intelligence and trust. Feelings and thoughts of logic, communication, and duty go with the color blue. This color can easily make you feel more well-spoken, smart, and efficient. Your Throat Chakra is the first of the chakras that is a completely spiritual chakra. An unhealthy Throat Chakra will cause you to have trouble speaking freely, staying focused, and paying attention when others are speaking. It may also cause you to fear being judged by other people. When this chakra is unhealthy, it can also cause physical ailments like tension headaches, stiffness in the shoulders and neck, problems with the thyroid gland, and excessive sore throats.

THE THIRD EYE CHAKRA – Deep knowledge and intuition lie in the Third Eye Chakra. This chakra is located directly in the center of your forehead. Its theme is 'to see.' Its corresponding color is indigo, and its element is light. This chakra controls your pituitary gland, the eyes, and the ears. The Solar Plexus Chakra is the balancing chakra. An unhealthy Third Eye Chakra will cause you to have trouble sleeping, including nightmares or night terrors. You might hallucinate or have other strange visions, and you will most likely suffer from headaches and will often be confused. Your sixth sense lies in your Third Eye Chakra, the sense allowing you to determine your feelings about other people and situations. When this chakra is unhealthy, you will feel disillusioned by life, or you may feel your feelings and thoughts are not really your own. In order to embrace your own intuition, your Third Eye Chakra must be healthy and fully functioning. All things passing between you and the outside world must go through this chakra, which acts as the bridge between you and the outside world. A clearly opened Third Eye Chakra will allow you to see what is real even if it is clouded by illusion and drama. If this chakra is unhealthy you will find it difficult to use your intuition, recall important facts, learn new skills, or even to trust your own inner voice. When the lower chakras are imbalanced, it will make the Third Eye Chakra imbalanced as well and can make you feel more introverted, judgmental, and dismissive toward other people. It can also make you feel depressed, anxious, and suffer from headaches and dizziness.

THE CROWN CHAKRA –The highest of the chakras inside your body is the Crown Chakra. It is where the source of the divine entity is found and is your connection to the spiritual world beyond you. This chakra is found at the top of your head, its color is white or violet, and no element corresponds with it. The Crown Chakra directly controls the cerebral cortex, which is responsible for personality and intelligence, gross motor skills and fine motor function, processing language, and the operation of the senses and the pineal gland, which is responsible for the regulation of all of the hormones in the body. Its theme is 'to understand,' and the Root Chakra balances it. If your Crown Chakra is unhealthy in any way you will have problems with your spirituality. You may deny the existence of any sort of higher power. You may become overly opinionated or feel as though you do not connect well with other people. You will probably struggle to understand spiritual concepts and you might even fear anything that has to do with spirituality and mysticism such as the occult or religion. You cannot access your higher powers if your Crown Chakra is not healthy. This can cause you to feel isolated or emotionally distressed. The colors of the Crown Chakra, violet and white, stand for oneness, spirituality, and meditation, as these are the ways to enable access to your Crown Chakra. It is possible to live with an unhealthy Crown Chakra, but you will never be able to feel truly spiritual or one with the universe.

The chart shows the colors corresponding to the main seven chakras. The names on the left side are the Sanskrit names for the chakras.

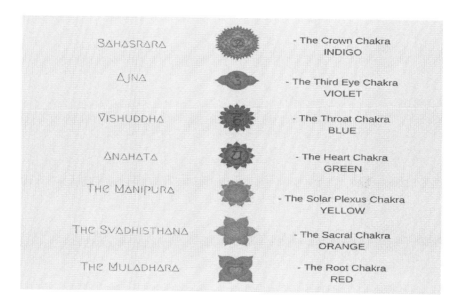

SAHASRARA		- The Crown Chakra INDIGO
AJNA		- The Third Eye Chakra VIOLET
VISHUDDHA		- The Throat Chakra BLUE
ANAHATA		- The Heart Chakra GREEN
THE MANIPURA		- The Solar Plexus Chakra YELLOW
THE SVADHISTHANA		- The Sacral Chakra ORANGE
THE MULADHARA		- The Root Chakra RED

THE CAUSAL CHAKRA– This chakra is also known as the Past Life Chakra or the Lunar Chakra. It is located three to four inches behind the back of your head, and the color of this chakra is white. You will receive information, inspiration, and messages related to intuition, love, and compassion through this chakra. The Causal Chakra activates and opens a gateway to the Angelic Kingdom. It will open strong communication to allow you to access information from the higher realms of the spiritual world.

When you receive this information, it will be distributed throughout the lower energy centers, filling your entire body. This chakra will help you explore the spirit world and higher wisdom better than would be readily available otherwise. This chakra will be open when your right brain is active, because it will help you to see the larger picture of the world using creativity and intuition.

THE SOUL STAR CHAKRA – This chakra, found about six inches above the top of your head and also known as the Solar Chakra, is the first of the transpersonal chakras, the ones surrounding your body on the stellar pathway around you. This chakra is closely aligned with the Crown Chakra, and it represents the spiritual, divine energy flowing through the universe. These two chakras are closely related because both deal with the spiritual forces of nature. But the Crown Chakra is more ego driven in that it will allow you to connect with and understand the spiritual world while remaining separate from it. The Soul Star Chakra drives you to become one with the universe through understanding and connecting with it. When your Soul Star Chakra is aligned with the remainder of your chakras, you will know your place in the universe through your renewed sense of purposefulness. If your Soul Star Chakra is spinning too rapidly, you will feel frivolous and restless, and you will find yourself searching for grounding. When this chakra is unhealthy or spinning too slowly, you will feel anxiety and a loss of purpose in life. The color of this chakra is white.

THE UNIVERSAL CHAKRA–Also known as the Galactic Chakra, this chakra is above the Soul Star Chakra and it is one of the iridescent colors, a mixture of silver, gold, and violet. This chakra is a channel for prophecy. It also connects you to the flow of energy in the universe, and through it, you can develop powerful abilities to heal. You will also be able to develop your psychic abilities further than ever before. You will receive extra-sensory perception, cosmic wisdom, and divine knowledge through this chakra. It will let you see past your body and mind and learn about human existence in its purest form, where you will be able to become fully aware of your role in the universe.

THE DIVINE GATEWAY CHAKRA – The final step in the chakras and in your ascension through them is the Divine Gateway Chakra, the chakra at the highest point of all of the chakras. It is the pinnacle of your system of chakras. When you activate and open this chakra, you can experience unhindered and free-flowing communication with the energies of the universe. This chakra is the gateway that allows you to explore all of the worlds beyond your consciousness. You will experience the deepest love, unity, and inner peace known to man. You will be happier and more successful when you are fully in touch with your deepest truths, and the Divine Gateway Chakra will help you to find and unlock them. This will mean you are truly connected to your true purpose and nature in life. If you have not been able to open and activate this chakra you might be feeling stuck in your present job, or you desire an accomplishment in life you just have not been able to achieve.

All of your chakras play an important role in your physical, mental, emotional, and spiritual health. A chakra more spiritual in nature will also assist you with your physical health because all of the health in your body is interdependent on one another. As the chakras spin and draw in energy, they also send out energy to your body, and this is what makes your body function at its peak capacity. The chakras are ever evolving while remaining rooted in their own particular function and position.

3

CHAPTER:
Reiki

Reiki is healing with energy, a form of alternative medicine. Reiki healers use hands-on healing with a technique called palm healing. The word is a combination of two words: the word 'rei,' which means divine, miraculous, and spiritual, and the word 'ki,' which means consciousness, vitality, and breath of life. Reiki is a subtle method of using energy to guide the life force in you.

All of the energy flowing through all living things is Reiki. The healers who practice this know everyone has the ability to heal themselves by connecting with their own energy and use it to strengthen themselves and others. Your energy, your ki, needs to be free-flowing and strong. When it is, your mind and body are in a positive state of being and health. If this energy is blocked or weak, you will experience feelings of emotional or physical imbalance.

The origins of Reiki date back to the late nineteenth century or the early part of the twentieth century, and they originated from the teachings of Japanese monks. The specific techniques and methods are drawn from the philosophies of several different practices of Asian healing. Reiki conceptualizes that diseases are caused by an imbalance of the vital energy of the body, and once those imbalances are corrected, the body will heal. This concept was widely believed in Western medicine up until the Middle Ages and is still used in Eastern medicine today.

Modern practitioners use this ancient concept of an inexhaustible source of energy healers can harness for healing the body. A master of the Reiki technique can use a process called attunements to teach other people how to master this powerful healing method. During a Reiki session, the patient lies down on a table while the healer places their hands on or hovering just over the patient. Energy will then flow down through the hands of the healer and into the patient. The basis behind the idea is that energy in the body will become blocked where there is an illness or an injury. The Reiki healing will remove the blocks and allow the energy to flow freely once again. There are several different health benefits associated with the practice of Reiki.

- Reiki can improve conditions and symptoms such as nausea, insomnia, tension, and headache.

- Reiki can be used to improve your mood by helping relieve your depression and anxiety.
- Reiki can help improve your quality of life by decreasing your levels of depression, increasing self-confidence, and improving sleep patterns, which helps you relax and give you inner peace and calm.
- Reiki can be used to treat depression by helping relieve your anxiety, depression, and physical pain. When your physical symptoms are improved your overall sense of good mood and well-being will also improve.
- Reiki helps reduce fatigue, anxiety, and pain in people with chronic or serious illnesses.

The practitioner might also use crystals to enhance the Reiki treatment. These might be placed around or on your body, or the healer might ask you to hold one in your hands. The crystals will have a calming effect on you, which will help intensify the effects of the healing. Crystals used might include aquamarine, tourmaline, topaz, moonstone, amethyst, or rose quartz.

Reiki can easily be used to heal the chakras and gets the energy flowing again so the entire body will benefit. When your energy is able to flow through your entire body unimpeded, your chakras will perform the way they were meant to perform. Every chakra plays a role in balancing some part of your life: spiritually, mentally, emotionally, or physically. The chakras inside your body can be affected by many things, from negative mental dialogue to a poor physical environment. A practitioner will use the techniques of Reiki to balance the chakras by removing the blockage preventing the energy from flowing freely through the body. They will clear out any blockages, balance the chakras, and repair imbalances in your aura.

When your energy is flowing freely and well-balanced, the energy of the spirit will be able to meet the energy of the body to contribute to the overall health of the body. Reiki can also help you prepare your mind to receive spiritual healing. Chakras can become unbalanced by negative energy received from other people, not paying attention to the needs of your inner self or getting your mind stuck in a manner of thinking that is not positive to the body. During the Reiki session, your mind is stilled while your body relaxes, and this will greatly improve your mental states. When you are able to find inner peace, you will be able to achieve the perfect state to meet guides to the spirit world and to hear your inner voice speaking to you.

Using Reiki to remove blocks of energy and rebalance the chakras can be a simple method for you to use. The healing practitioner can work on one chakra at a time or on all of your internal chakras. Once they have rebalanced your chakras, it will be easy to periodically rebalance them and clear out any blockages before they become major problems.

4
CHAPTER:
Self-Healing Your Chakras

Energy radiates from everything in the universe. Between the tiniest blade of grass and the tallest mountain, between the largest ocean and all of the cells in your body, energy flows. Your cells give off energy in various ways, and the different cells in your body give off different types of energy depending on what their function is and where they are located. There are several different channels located in specific areas of the body allowing energy to flow out and in at a constant pace. These are your chakras.

The chakras spin in a clockwise direction to move energy out of your body and counterclockwise to pull energy into your body. The current state of the individual chakra will determine the direction the energy will flow through your body. The opening and closing of the chakras are part of your body's internal defense mechanism. If you have a negative experience, the chakra associated with that feeling will close so it can block out that negative energy. You can close off a chakra by holding on to certain thoughts and feelings, which will cause the chakra to close to protect itself. When you heal your chakras and open them again, the energy is once again able to flow freely, and your energy levels will soon return to normal. Since every chakra is attached to a certain part of the nervous system and the endocrine system in your body, a closed chakra could lead to an energy deficiency, which might cause a serious physical ailment if left for too long.

All of your chakras are equally important to your body in terms of balancing and flowing energy levels. An ideal situation is when all seven of your internal chakras are balanced, open, healed, and spinning at the proper frequency. Your body will find ways to move energy around. So, if one of your chakras is closed, the one next to it or its balancing chakra will work overtime to compensate for the deficiency. Your body wants a balance of energy, so it will find ways to make this happen. If one chakra is underperforming, it will cause another to overperform, and this will naturally upset the balance of the chakras in your body. The first step is being able to recognize when your chakras are imbalanced, because overperforming is just as bad for your body as underperforming. Here are the feelings you might experience when any of your internal chakras are underactive or overactive:

Root Chakra

Underactive – fearful of abandonment, codependent, lacking a sense of being at home or secure anywhere, unable to get into one's body

Overactive – Resistant to change, insecure, nervous, materialistic or greedy, ungrounded, fearful

Physical Symptoms of Imbalance – Restlessness, unhealthy weight (either obesity or eating disorder), inability to sit still, constipation, cramps, fatigue or sluggishness

Associated Organs and Endocrine Glands – Spine, blood, adrenal glands, and reproductive organs

Sacral Chakra

Underactive – lacking self-esteem or self-worth, unemotional, stiff, closed off to others, possibly in an abusive relationship

Overactive – very quick to attach and invest in others, moody, overemotional, attracted to drama, lacking personal boundaries

Physical Symptoms of Imbalance – Urinary issues, kidney pain or infection, lower back pain or stiffness, infertility, impotence

Associated Organs and Endocrine Glands – Kidneys and reproductive organs: ovaries, testes, and uterus

Solar Plexus Chakra

Underactive – Lacking self-control, timid, passive, indecisive

Overactive – Angry, aggressive, domineering, perfectionist or overly critical of oneself or others

Physical Symptoms of Imbalance – Eating disorders; asthma or other respiratory ailments; ulcers, gas, nausea, or other digestive problems; nerve pain or fibromyalgia; infection in the liver or kidneys; other organ problems

Associated Organs and Endocrine Glands – Digestive system (stomach and intestines), central nervous system, liver, pancreas, metabolic system

Heart Chakra

Underactive – Unable or unwilling to open up to others, lonely, cold, distant, grudgeful

Overactive – Willing to say yes to everything, lacking a sense of self in a relationship, loving in a clingy, suffocating way, lacking boundaries, letting everyone in

Physical Symptoms of Imbalance – Asthma or other respiratory ailments, breast cancer, poor circulation or numbness, heart and circulatory problems (heart palpitations, high blood pressure, and heart attack), stiff joints or joint problems in the hands

Associated Organs and Endocrine Glands – Heart, lungs, thymus gland and immune system, breasts, arms, hands

Throat Chakra

Underactive – Having difficulty speaking the truth, introverted, shy, and unable to express needs

Overactive – verbally abusive, unable to listen, overly talkative, highly critical, condescending

Physical Symptoms of Imbalance – Earaches or infection, hoarseness or laryngitis, stiffness or soreness in the neck or shoulders, sore throat, dental issues or TMJ, thyroid issues

Associated Organs and Endocrine Glands – Neck, throat, thyroid, shoulders, ears, and mouth

Third Eye Chakra

Underactive – Closed off to new ideas, disconnected or distrustful of inner voice, rigid in thinking, too reliant on authority, anxious, clinging to the past and fearful of the future

Overactive – Lacking good judgment, unable to focus, out of touch with reality, prone to hallucinations

Physical Symptoms of Imbalance – Headaches or migraines, insomnia or sleep disorders, vision problems, seizures, nightmares (though this isn't a physical symptom per se; it is a common occurrence)

Associated Organs and Endocrine Glands – Eyes, brow, pituitary, base of skull, biorhythms

Crown Chakra

Underactive – Unable to set or maintain goals, not very open to spirituality, lacking direction

Overactive – Heedless of bodily needs, addicted to spirituality, having difficulty controlling emotions

Physical Symptoms of Imbalance – Nerve pain, mental fog, dizziness, neurological disorders, confusion, schizophrenia or other mental disorders

Associated Organs and Endocrine Glands – Hypothalamus, pituitary and pineal glands, cerebral cortex, brain, central nervous system

There are several different methods that you can use for healing and balancing your chakras.

MEDITATION – It is often easier to focus on the body as a whole than to try working on each chakra individually. This is especially true if you are just learning to work on your chakras. You can use meditation as an access point to any chakra you want to focus on. When you have spent enough time healing your chakras with meditation, then you will become better at isolating one and focusing on it. You will do best in a quiet place where you can have at least thirty minutes alone. Sit comfortably and let yourself relax. Sit up straight but do not let your body be tense or rigid. Breathe in and out steadily and slowly. Imagine each of the seven internal chakras in your mind. Picture them as healthy and open with energy flowing through them at a proper rate. Set your focus on each chakra for at least several minutes. Use any meditation tools or guided meditation to help you meditate.

CRYSTALS AND STONES – Crystals and stones come in many colors, and it is easy to find ones you can use to heal and balance your chakras. Chapter Five will cover more of this information for you. You can use one single crystal or a different color for every chakra. The easiest way to balance your chakras using crystals is to lie down and set a crystal on your body at a point corresponding with a chakra. Be sure to lie still for at least ten minutes while you allow the crystals to do their work.

ESSENTIAL OILS – There are different essential oils corresponding to each of the internal chakras. According Healthcare America the following essential oils correspond to each chakra:

Root -Patchouli Essential Oil encourages stimulation in this center while, encouraging balance. It is also said to help stimulate the Sacral Chakra (second chakra). Another suggestion would be to use Cypress essential oil

Sacral Chakra - Neroli Essential Oil will bring balance here and will also assist in stimulating the Heart Chakra. Another essential oil suggestion would be Ylang Ylang

Solar Plexus - Pine Essential Oil will bring benefit to the Solar Plexus while again adding benefits for the Heart Chakra. An alternative suggestion would be to use Ginger.

Heart Chakra - Rosewood or Rose Essential Oil will help release feelings of constriction and help maintain a healthy aura. An alternative oil to use would be Jasmine

Throat Chakra – Lavender Essential Oil- Can help heal feelings of being withdrawn and encourages expanded awareness and communication. Another oil suggestion would be Roman Chamomile

Third Eye Chakra - Sandalwood Essential Oil will help with inner awareness allowing you to engage with higher consciousness. An alternative could be Rosemary

Crown Chakra - Lime Essential Oil, is useful in enhancing perception and can assist with energetic cord cutting. An alternative oil could be Frankincense.

When you use essential oils on your skin, you will need to add a few drops of carrier oil because essential oil by itself is too potent to put on your skin. Using a diffuser, put in several drops of the essential oil of your choice and inhale the scent while you sit peacefully or meditate. You can also rub the essential oil with carrier oil between your palms and then rub it on the area of the body that the chakra is connected to.

YOGA – Yoga poses are an amazing way to open and balance the chakras. They will promote the flow of energy in your body. The postures and movements found in yoga are known to expel negative energy and unblock the chakras. They also encourage positive energy to flow into the person.

COLOR – Since each of the chakras has its own corresponding color, you can easily use color to heal and balance your chakras. Certain colors make people feel certain feelings, and your emotions and moods will be affected by certain colors. If you need to target one specific chakra, you should wear the colors corresponding with that chakra. You can also surround yourself with furnishings and décor in the color scheme of the chakras you feel need the most healing.

MASSAGE – By massaging the area where the chakra is located, you will help to balance it.

AFFIRMATIONS – This is a powerful yet simple way to clear and balance your chakras. You will simply chant or meditate on positive statements, such as the theme of the chakra you are trying to heal. Positive statements hold power to heal and strengthen damaged parts of your body. When you use them properly, you are able to give your complete attention to a part of yourself needing assistance.

Since the five remaining chakras are outside of your body, you will need to use meditation in order to open them to complete your chakra balancing. Whichever method you choose to heal your chakras, or whether you choose to use them all, your chakras will support you best when they are balanced and healthy.

5

CHAPTER:
Crystal Therapy to Heal the Chakras

You can balance your chakras with crystals so that the energy centers holding your life force will work more efficiently. You can use one single crystal or several crystals in every color of the rainbow, and they can be used to heal and balance your chakras. Your chakras connect your mind and body to your spirit and emotions. If your chakras become unhealthy or unbalanced, diseases and illnesses of the body, mind, and spirit will happen as a result. Your chakras can become closed or blocked for many different reasons, including emotional upsets, illnesses, or problems with karma. Sometimes there are issues that began in childhood events or in past lives causing chakra imbalances or closures. When you use crystals, they will vibrate at the exact frequency of the chakra and will help heal it.

The easiest way to align all of the chakras at once is to lie down with a crystal lying over each of the chakras. You will want to choose a crystal whose color corresponds to the color of that chakra. You will want to lie completely still for at least ten minutes with each crystal in place over the chakra it corresponds to and focus on keeping your breathing deep and steady. Place the crystal for the Root Chakra just beneath the Root Chakra– in between the tops of your legs– and place the crystal for the Crown Chakra on the top of your head. Place the rest of the crystals on your body at the chakra they correspond with. Remember to clean your crystals well after you use them. As a reminder, the points below show the colors of the crystals corresponding with the colors of the chakras.

- **Root Chakra** – black or red crystal
- **Sacral Chakra** – orange or blue-green crystal
- **Solar Plexus Chakra** – yellow or gold crystal
- **Heart Chakra** – green or pink crystal
- **Throat Chakra** – blue crystal
- **Third Eye Chakra** – violet or purple crystal
- **Crown Chakra** – white or violet crystal

When you are using crystals to heal your chakras, you will lie flat on your back facing up. Imagine each of the chakras as a glowing wheel as it rapidly spins while rotating in a clockwise direction. Visually imagine the energy of the crystals blending and mixing with the unique colors of every chakra. You will use your chakras to receive and transmit spiritual, emotional, and physical energy. Your ideal state of being is to have all your chakra centers vitalized, balanced, and clear to give your body optimal well-being. The following list will show you which stones to use with each of your chakras, as well as a reminder of what energies correspond to each chakra:

Root Chakra – The focus of its energy is security, free will, physical energy, grounding, and stability. The crystals used for this chakra are spinel, garnet, zircon, hematite, smoky quartz, black obsidian, and black tourmaline.

Sacral Chakra – The focus of its energy is intuition, emotion, desire, healing, creativity, and reproduction and sexuality. The crystals used for this chakra are imperial topaz, carnelian, vanadinite, copper, blue-green turquoise, blue-green fluorite, and orange calcite.

Solar Plexus Chakra – Its energy is protection, ambition, personal power, and intellect. The crystals for this chakra are gold tiger eye, citrine, yellow apatite, amber, golden calcite, and yellow jasper.

Heart Chakra – The focus of its energy is emotional balance, love, compassion, and universal consciousness. The crystals for this chakra are jade, rose quartz, malachite, cobaltian calcite, green aventurine, pink danburite, watermelon tourmaline, lepidolite, pink tourmaline, rosasite, and vesuvianite.

Throat Chakra – The focus of its energy is divine guidance, expression, and communication. The crystals for this chakra are aquamarine, sodalite, amazonite, blue calcite, blue turquoise, chrysocolla, blue kyanite, angelate, celestite, and blue chalcedony.

Third Eye Chakra – The focus of its energy is light, psychic power, intuition, and spiritual awareness. The crystals for this chakra are tanzanite, lapis lazuli, and azurite.

Crown Chakra – Its energy is perfection, energy, enlightenment, and cosmic consciousness. The crystals for this chakra are selenite, amethyst, white Howlite, apophyllite, white danburite, diamond, white topaz, quartz crystal, and white hemimorphite.

As you become more familiar with crystals and the energies around and within you, you will begin to incorporate this awareness into different aspects of your consciousness and your life. Studying and working with crystals and with your chakras will help you become aware of the energy existing within your spirit, mind, and body.

6

CHAPTER:
Meditation for Healing the Chakras

Any type of meditation can be used to support your chakras, as meditation will open and balance your chakras. The very act of meditation brings quiet and calm to your mind and body, which is the best state for the chakras to begin to relax and heal. It helps to clear away mental and emotional blockages that will eventually cause physical damage to your body. The field of human energy is open and constantly moving. When you use meditation to cleanse your chakras of imbalances, you release blocked energy and allow it to flow freely again.

You will want to use chakra specific meditations, so you are able to directly affect the specific chakra you want to work on. This will bring balance and health to all of the spiritual, mental, emotional, and physical aspects associated with that chakra. You will be able to open the chakras spiritually and energetically. One of the best features of guided meditation for chakras is that using the proper words will release the blockage of a specific chakra. Guided meditations are helpful when they are used to heal your chakras, and they will quite often have an immediate effect on your personal mood and vibration. The words of the meditation are soothing enough to heal your body, powerful enough to energize your spirit, and direct enough to re-program your mind.

There are affirmations for each chakra that can be used as guided meditations. The best way to use affirmations is to repeat the statements as a form of meditation while feeling the positive emotion associated with that affirmation. Guided meditations can be used daily or anytime you feel your chakras might need an extra bit of healing. Guided meditations will only be effective if phrased in the present tense. You will use the theme words corresponding to each chakra to energize the center while healing any imbalances in the energy of the chakras. This will also heal any associated emotional, physical, or mental problems related to that particular chakra. You can also create affirmations for guided meditation by using any of the keywords correlating to any of the chakras. Just keep in mind the statements you use in your meditations should be self-affirming, self-empowering, and positive statements serving to lift you up and energize and inspire you.

Simply choose one of these affirmations and repeat it over and over as a meditation, or you can create a phrase of your own.

Guided Meditations for the Root Chakra

I am

I have

I live

Use the theme words corresponding with the Root Chakra to create positive and uplifting statements:

I am living life to the fullest

I am located exactly where I want to be right now

I am protected, safe, and secure

I am supported and safe in my body

I have a healthy strong body

I have a strong foundation

I have prosperity and abundance

I have safety and support from the earth

I have self-control

I have strength and courage

I live a life supported by the universe

I live a life that is protected and nurtured

I remain at peace with my surroundings

I stay connected to the Earth and well-grounded

I have a right to be here

Guided Meditations for the Sacral Chakra

I sense

I want

I feel

Use the theme words corresponding with the Sacral Chakra to create positive and uplifting statements:

I want to enjoy my body

I sense my deeper connection to my body and the Earth

I want a natural sense of joy

I feel my creative expression

I feel sensual in my being

I feel nurtured and protected

I want to flow with ease and grace

I want to trust my own intuition

I feel a sense of abundance

I feel clear and free

I want to release those things that do not serve me

I want to express myself with ease

I feel safe and secure

I feel passion and joy

I sense my intuitive senses are now awake

Guided Meditations for the Solar Plexus Chakra

I act

I think

I will

Use the theme words corresponding with the Solar Plexus Chakra to create positive and uplifting statements:

I am a responsible human being

I am in control of my life

I am focused and empowered

I will use my personal power for good things

I will persevere through uncertainty

I am ambitious and self-motivated

I act like a responsible person

I will harness the power of my own will

I will be full of personal power and courage

I act relaxed in situations that are challenging

I will commit myself to my goals

I will treat myself with respect

I act in a self-motivated manner

I will fully step into my power

I will achieve my goals successfully

Guided Meditations for the Heart Chakra

I receive

I give

I love

Use the theme words corresponding with the Heart Chakra to create positive and uplifting statements:

I love myself and others unconditionally

I love my life and all that it brings to me

I love myself enough to forgive myself when needed

I receive and give love easily

I accept and love the person I am now

I love the energy of the universe flowing through my body

Love is the language I speak to others

Love is a magnificent force in my life

I am open to knowing wonderful peace and joy in my life

I receive the gifts that I am given by the people who love me

I give compassion and love to all people of the Earth

Love flows through my being to other people

I receive compassion and acceptance from the people in my life

I am open to receiving strength from the Higher Power

My heart is connected to others by love

Guided Meditation for the Throat Chakra

I express

I listen

I speak

Use the theme words corresponding with the Throat Chakra to create positive and uplifting statements:

I listen to the truth within me

I speak the truth as my heart feels it

My voice is unique and I speak what I think

I express love and gratitude toward life

I express my thoughts with confidence and clarity

My voice is my ally and my friend

I express my feelings with honesty and truth

I speak to others with kindness

My voice has the power to say what I need to say

I listen to others because their words are important to me

I listen to the Higher Power and what it says to me

My voice is my own and I will use it

I listen without judgment when others speak to me

I listen to others with compassion and empathy

My voice is my instrument to spread love and peace in the world

Guided Meditations for the Third Eye Chakra

I imagine

I envision

I see

Use the theme words corresponding with the Third Eye Chakra to create positive and uplifting statements:

I see my imagination open to all possibilities

I see beyond illusions to the truth of the matter

I envision a clear path toward my goals

I imagine a healthy spirit, mind, and body

I envision my mind focused and clear

I imagine my mind filled with guidance and wisdom

I envision a bright and positive future filled with hope

I imagine my life going exactly the way it should

I envision a peaceful world well filled with joy and love

I imagine the goodness in others and try to see it

I am imaginative and insightful

I see great possibilities in my future life

I see when things are going well in my world

I envision my inner knowing accepting my psychic potential

I see the light of my higher mind illuminating my life

Guided Meditation for the Crown Chakra

I am

I know

I understand

Use the theme words corresponding with the Crown Chakra to create positive and uplifting statements:

I am able to see the bigger picture of life

I know there is goodness in all things

I know I have a higher purpose and it will be fulfilled

I am faithful that everything will turn out well

I understand there is a divine and natural order to the world

I am seeking wisdom and understanding from my life experiences

I am open to the wisdom of the universe

I know that everything is good in my world

I am open to receiving Divine Energy from the Higher Power

I understand that I am a powerful force in my own life

I am open to receive goodness and abundance from the universe

I am connected to the greater world with love

I am seeking healing and balance from the power of life

I am healing on all levels of my being

I understand the purity of love and life

The only way to open and balance the top five chakras is through meditation, since they lie outside of the physical body. There is a wonderful method for opening them through meditation. Sit down where you can be comfortable and undisturbed. You will need to sit with your back straight and your spine long and strong. Let your breath fill your body from the top of your head down to your feet. Feel the breath seeping from your feet and into the floor below you. Keep your spine straight but let the muscles of your back relax. Picture in your mind a golden orb above your head, floating freely. This is the Divine Gateway you are opening to allow strength and energy from the universe to flow through you. Just below the Divine Gateway is the Universal Chakra, which begins to open and energize with the golden light flowing toward you from the divine Gateway. Next in line is the Soul Star Chakra, which is the representation of your higher self. Feel it begin to open and energize as the golden light continues to flow from the universe toward you, opening and energizing your higher chakras. Your higher mind, your Causal Chakra, begins to feel the effect of the streaming light from the universe as it begins opening to allow the golden light to flow into the chakras in your body. Allow the golden light to flow into you and down through the seven chakras of the body. Feel it continue to flow through your feet and down into you Earth Star Chakra. Now the glowing golden light from the universe has opened and energized all of your chakras, allowing you to think and feel on a higher plane than ever before.

You can use your guided meditations in order from the Root Chakra to the Crown Chakra and then back down. Or you can use them in no particular order to balance and heal any of your chakras that might need a little more attention at the moment. Your meditations can be done at any time of the day; find a time and a place that feels relaxing and restful to meditate and to repeat the affirmations as long as you feel the need to. More frequent meditation will give you faster balancing and healing of your chakras. Meditation offers great power for healing, so use it as often as possible.

7
CHAPTER:
Yoga for Healing the Chakras

U sing yoga poses to balance your chakras will enable you to become more aware of the subtle energy system of your body and how energy flows through your body. Perfect health will come to you when your chakras are balanced and open. Sometimes your energy becomes stuck in one or more particular chakras. When performing yoga poses, you focus on every energy center in your body, which allows you to open your chakras and bring balance to them so your spirit, mind, and body will once again be whole. Balance is important for your life force, your energy, to flow freely through your body.

Besides being a physical movement awakening the body, you can practice yoga poses without really thinking about them, so your mind is free to relax. This will help bring positive energy to and through your centers of energy in your subtle body. Here are some of the many yoga poses that can be used to open, balance, and heal your chakras:

Root Chakra

Tree pose will keep your Root Chakra balanced and open. This pose will give you feelings of security, stability, and alertness. The Root Chakra influences your survival instincts and family ties, which are so important in today's world. This chakra will also govern how much of a sense of belonging you have with the world around you and how guarded you are.

To do the tree pose, stand perfectly straight and tall with your arms at the side of your body. Bend your right knee slightly and place the bottom of your right foot firmly high up on the thigh of your left leg. Make sure the sole of your foot is placed firmly and flat on the inside of your left thigh. Your left leg will need to be kept completely steady and straight, and it is important for you to remain as balanced and still as possible while you are doing this pose.

Inhale deeply and raise both of your arms over your head and hold your palms together. Fix your gaze on some distant object and look straight ahead with an unwavering gaze. Keep your spine straight and your body firm but not too rigid. Breathe deeply while you hold the pose for a few minutes, then relax and repeat the entire routine with your left leg.

It is important when doing this pose that the bottom of your foot is placed on the thigh above your knee, or below if necessary, for good balance. The sole of the foot must never be placed beside you, because this would put improper pressure on your knee. If holding your arms over your head is too difficult, then put your palms together in front of your chest.

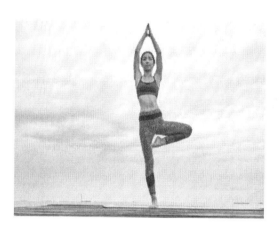

Sacral Chakra

Your Sacral Chakra governs your lower abdomen and your sexuality. If your Sacral Chakra is healthy, you will enjoy your sexual energy without feeling guilty about possessing it. This will allow you to become comfortable in your intimate relationships and to be passionate but not overly needy or demanding. When your Sacral Chakra is not active enough, you will lose interest in relationships and be void of emotions. When it is too active, then you will be constantly emotional and sensitive.

The Goddess Pose will keep your Sacral Chakra healthy and open and will stimulate emotional creativity and stability. This pose will also help enhance sexual energy and fertility while bringing balance to your chakra. Let your arms hang beside your body with your hands on your hips. Place your feet about four feet apart on the floor and turn your toes outward slightly. Breathe deeply and bend your knees but do not let them stick out beyond your toes. Squat until your hips are bent well and your thighs are held parallel to the floor. You may not be able to squat this far at first, but that is the ultimate goal. While in the squat stretch your arms out to your sides at the same height as your shoulders with your palms facing downward, and then bring your palms together in front of your chest, keeping your forearms bent at a ninety-degree angle. Keep your tailbone tucked under your body and gaze forward. Hold this pose for around thirty seconds before you release it.

Solar Plexus Chakra

A Solar Plexus Chakra that is open and healthy will give you a great feeling of dignity and a sense of being in control over things. If your Solar Plexus chakra is closed or unhealthy, you will suffer from feelings of indecisiveness and passivity. If this chakra is overactive, it will lead you to become aggressive and overbearing.

The boat pose will keep your Solar Plexus Chakra healthy and open to a proper level. This pose will give you a wonderful boost to your confidence and an increased sense of self-esteem. Lie on your back flat on the floor and place your arms beside your body and keep your feet together. Take in a deep breath and when you exhale, lift your feet up off the floor and your chest raised while you stretch your arms toward your feet. Keep your fingers, toes, and eyes in a perfectly straight line. Your abdominal muscles will contract and the area under your belly button should begin to stretch. Keep breathing deeply and normally as much as possible while you maintain the pose. Exhale when you release the pose.

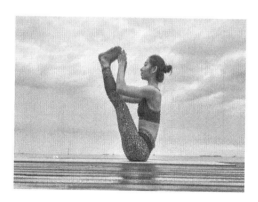

Heart Chakra

When your Heart Chakra is open and healthy, you will enjoy feelings of warmth, friendliness, and compassion toward others. You will be closed up, cold, and unfriendly if this chakra is not active. But if this chakra is too active you could inadvertently appear to be selfish because you will suffocate people with too much love. That is why it is vital you keep your Heart Chakra spinning just right.

The Camel Pose will relieve stress in your mind and body. Put your hands on your hips while you kneel on the floor or on a mat. Keep your lower legs flat on the floor with the soles of your feet facing the ceiling. Your knees and shoulders need to stay in a straight line. Inhale deeply and pull your tailbone in toward your pelvis. You will feel a gentle pulling sensation at your belly button. Arch your back and lay the palms of your hands over your feet while keeping your arms straight. Keep your neck relaxed so it will not feel strained. Hold this pose for thirty to sixty seconds before you gently release it.

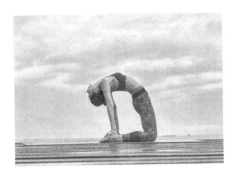

Throat Chakra

Your Throat Chakra helps you to speak clearly. When this chakra is healthy and well-balanced, you will be able to easily express yourself, and you will use your creativity to be more expressive. If your Throat Chakra is unbalanced or blocked, you will most likely be shy and speak less. If your Throat Chakra is totally blocked, you will regularly feel the need to lie to other people. If your chakra is too active, you might repel some people because you will listen less than you need to, and you will talk way too much.

A pose to keep your Throat Chakra open and healthy is the shoulder stand. It begins with you lying flat on the floor on your back with your legs together and your arms at your sides. With one quick movement lift your legs, buttocks, and back and let your elbows hold up your lower body so your body is literally standing on the lower part of your body. Keep your legs firm and hold this pose for around thirty to sixty seconds. Breathe deeply while you are in the pose.

Third Eye Chakra

You will dream regularly when the Third Eye Chakra is open and healthy. You will also possess an amazing intuition and have a good sixth sense. If you do not have an active Third

Eye, you will likely allow other people to make decisions you should be making for yourself, and you might be easily confused and rely on misleading information. If this chakra is overactive it will cause you to live in a world of imagination and dreams.

The pose to keep the Third Eye chakra opened and balanced works well when practiced regularly. It will help you develop your instincts and strengthen your intuition. Your Third Eye Chakra governs the functions of the rest of the chakras and it is very important that you keep it balanced.

Cross your legs while sitting on your bottom. Lay your hands on your knees with your fingers facing up and your thumb and index finger touching. Keep your spine firm and straight but not too stiff. Balance your spine on top of your pelvis and do not lean either forward or backward. Exhale slowly and let your shoulders relax, and then inhale deeply and lift your spine. Relax your body and keep your eyes closed. Keep breathing deeply and slowly while you hold the pose for a few minutes before releasing it.

Crown Chakra

Your Crown Chakra is the one responsible for your spirituality. It will increase your personal wisdom and make sure you become one in harmony with the universe around you. When your Crown Chakra is open you will be more aware of and open to the world around you and your connection with it. It will also help you to become more aware of yourself. Preconceived prejudices and notions you have will completely disappear.

When your Crown Chakra is underactive, you will not be spiritually open and aware, and you may suffer from rigid beliefs and stiff thoughts. If your Crown Chakra is too active, you will tend to over-analyze everything, and you will probably be overly spiritual. You may forget to attend to your worldly needs like food, water, and shelter.

Balance your Crown Chakra through meditation. Sit comfortably on the floor and cross your legs in front of you with your hands resting gently on your stomach or your knees. Begin to meditate with your eyes closed and your mind concentrating on your Crown Chakra. Think about all this chakra means to the energy level in your body and mind. Chant the sound "om" softly and clearly. Keep your mind and the body relaxed while keeping all of your focus on your Crown Chakra. You will need to meditate for at least ten minutes.

Do not do this meditation until after your Root Chakra has been opened and is strong and well-balanced, as it provides a strong foundation for the Crown Chakra Your Crown Chakra should be the last one to get attention.

Using yoga poses is one of the easiest ways to keep your chakras healthy and balanced. You can do some sort of yoga pose every day if you want. Keeping your chakras open and balanced is important for keeping your body and mind in

good health. This will enable you to live your life to the fullest and enjoy every minute of being alive.

8

CHAPTER:
Unicorns

Unicorns are mythical creatures that hold a place in people's hearts and have done so for generations. They capture the imagination of children, poets, artists, and writers with their graceful purity. Unicorns are transcendent creatures thought to exist on a higher plane in other dimensions. Their magic gives off very high vibrational energies as they have a fully awakened third eye chakra. It is this chakra that sends off a spiraling white light some see or depict as a horn. Even though they choose to ascend as the proud majestic horse, their energies as well as light, match those of other ascended masters. These very high vibrational energies can help to cleanse our lower vibrations. Their light and energy realign the body, mind, and soul to bring about connectedness as well as balance.

Unicorns Spiritual Meanings

The unicorn has been a prominent feature in modern culture appearing in many spiritual traditions even in ancient times. These traditions are not limited to one part of the globe or a specific culture, they are utilized through every part from east to west. They are known as mystical creatures for a reason and have different mystical meanings:

Freedom

Unicorns are creatures that would rather risk death than be captured or held in any kind of captivity. They are a symbol of freedom, of letting go of those self-imposed prison cells that hold a person back from reaching their full potential.

Fear of failing, thinking you are not good enough or having a negative self-image holds one back from achieving great things. If a person can overcome the mental blocks, they put in their way, they will be able to accomplish anything.

To break these bonds and shackles that are limiting you, you need to tune in to the energies of the unicorn. Call upon them to liberate you from your self-imposed mental blocks.

Healing

A unicorn is full of a pure magic light which makes them natural healers. They are believed to be able to heal both emotional and physical pain with their tears. Aligning with their healing powers will help to heal the wounds that ache inside and out. They will help you to overcome anger and put you onto the path of forgiving those who have hurt you.

They can also open up your spirit to let in more love. They can help you be more creative, accepting that you deserve to be loved and fill your life with abundance.

Strength/Courage

Unicorns are fearless and will charge into battle or push the boundaries of their inner strength. If you are feeling alone, discouraged, or fearful, these noble creatures are there to bring you comfort, support and offer strength. They will guide you to open up and find your own courage to tackle any obstacles that may be blocking your path.

As they are also creatures that inspire us, they will encourage you to reach higher and move out of your comfort zone. They may be gentle, kind, and peaceful, but unicorns can also be fierce when defending what they need to defend. Draw on that strength and align it with your own for that bit of extra power you may need.

Wisdom

Unicorns are ancient creatures that have lived through worlds. They have wisdom beyond that of which you could even begin to imagine. When you are feeling in need of enlightenment and are stuck on a problem, or need to raise your vibrations, tap into the unicorn's wisdom.

They will help you overcome the difficulties of today, release the baggage of the past that is holding you back so you can fly easily into tomorrow. To release negativity, call upon them to help you purge self-doubt and gain inner wisdom as you open your soul.

Connection to Unicorns Through the Chakras

Unicorns can open a person's third eye to give one foresight and a greater understanding of the world around us. It can also allow us to have a greatest sense of self in that we can better feel what is out of sorts within us.

Unicorns are associated with the heart chakra, which is the fourth chakra. It is through the heart chakra that they can help a person open up to accept love, hope, friendship, and also give it back, unconditionally. The assistance of a unicorn can also be instrumental in opening and realigning the necessary outer chakras: The Soul Star Chakra, the Causal Chakra, and the Earth Star Chakra in particular.

You can connect to the unicorn through reiki, meditation, and crystals.

Getting in Touch With Your Unicorn Guide

Meditation is the best way to get in touch with your unicorn guide. If you struggle on your own in the beginning, you can try guided meditation.

Follow these simple steps to use meditation to get in touch with your unicorn guide and open your chakras:

- Set aside time in your day to meditate. Find a quiet place where you will not be disturbed.

- The heart chakra is associated with green. Wear green clothing and surround yourself with the color to ensure you draw in the correct energy.

- Place a comfortable mat on the floor and light a candle. If you are spiritual, you will want to honor the days of the week with their color candle.

  - Monday is a silver, white, or grey candle.
  - Tuesday is a red candle.
  - Wednesday is a purple candle.
  - Thursday is a blue candle.
  - Friday is a green candle.
  - Saturday is a black candle.
  - Sunday is a yellow candle (or a gold candle).

- Start your meditation by connecting with the earth and feeling yourself creating roots into the earth from your feet.

- Call upon an angel to keep you safe from negative energy that you may or may not be aware of.
- Visualize your intentions and softly say them to the universe.
- Keep your mind centered on your fourth chakra as you open a green light.
- Pull that light into your center and let it fill your heart as you allow the green to slowly spin, weaving into a ball of shimmering light.
- Visualize the light growing into a great shimmering white light ascending upon you that materializes into a unicorn.
- Connect with your unicorn and align yourself with its energies as you ask it to light your chakras to bring them into balance.
- Feel the energy flow through you as you picture a warm golden light that fills you from your feet to the tip of your head. Lighting up each of your chakras as it slowly ascends through your body.
- Once the light has filled you allow the energy to connect with your soul and guide it to your heart chakra.
- Allow the light in as you softly chant "I open my heart to love and accept that I am worthy of it in abundance."

- Feel the warmth of the unicorns love and accept it as it accepts the love you give unconditionally in return.
- Picture the light turning to green as you fill your heart with love.
- Breath in the green light and breath out letting the light become one once again with the great white light of the unicorn.
- Feel the connection as you float up realign with the soul star and sun star.
- Let go of the baggage of the past in this life and any that you may have lived before.
- Relax, breathe and let the energy surround you, drawing you deeper into the light until all the tension has left your body.
- Slowly allow yourself to float back to the present as you thank your unicorn for its love, guidance, and light.

- Thank your angel that kept you safe and protected you.

- Breath in the green light and center it with your fourth chakra.

- Slowly breath out and open your eyes.

Connecting to Unicorn Energy With Crystals

Crystals, like unicorns, are also from the earth and because of their great energetic properties, they can raise a person's vibrations. Some crystals resonate well with the vibrations of unicorns to help you connect with their energy.

You can use the following crystals to attune to the realm of the unicorns and connect to their energy.

Lepidolite

Lepidolite is a beautiful lavender colored crystal. It has a lovely sparkle to it that makes it bring out the love in a person. This crystal brings joy to a person's heart, opening it up and letting the love flow. It helps to center your vision to look within and realize how wonderful you are. Using this crystal will show you that you are worthy of receiving love and accepting all the good around you.

It is also a crystal that attracts love, loyalty, and lasting friendships. It is the unicorn of crystals. It embodies their love, kindness, and gentleness.

Apophyllite

The apophyllite crystal is used in meditation to help you transcend to other realms or worlds including that of the unicorns. It is a beautiful gem that is the color of starlight on a clear night sky. It has pyramid type tips that make it look like a little star and it sparkles like magic in the sunlight.

It is not hard to see why this little gem can help you reach interaction with unicorn energy.

Peridot

The peridot is a clear yellow-green stone that has a calm comforting vibration. It embodies all that is mother nature. It embraces the essence of the trees, flowers, herbs, and flows with the seasons. This helps a person to become more aware and connected harmoniously to the earth.

Once you have strengthened this connection, you can form a stronger bond with the vibration energies of the unicorn. They too are in complete harmony with the earth. The peridot stone allows you to connect with the peace and wisdom of the unicorn. It allows a person to gain emotional, physical, and mental health for a healthier lifestyle.

It is also the stone to use if you are looking to gain more inspiration or need to feel that you are connected.

Golden Labradorite

You only have to look at this crystal to be drawn into the mystical energies that surround it. Just like the mystical unicorn, it holds you spellbound with a need to reach out and touch it. It is a clear crystal that sparkles with a hypnotic golden center.

It holds the magic of creativity, clear thinking, a deeper awareness, and heart health. To tap into the magical energies of the unicorn and open up your inner voice, you should use the golden labradorite.

There are a few legends that surround these rare gems. One such legend tells that the northern lights were once trapped within the labradorite rocks. One day a warrior came upon these rocks striking them with his spear freeing them. However, he did not get all the rocks. To this day there are rocks that still hold parts of the northern lights within them giving them their luminous beauty.

Blue Lace Agate

If you need confidence and an increased ability to communicate with ease, then use blue lace agate. This crystal helps you tap into the unicorn's strength and confidence. It has a soothing quality about it just like the quiet strength of the unicorn. It will open up your inner strength, help you to keep a calm, cool, level head and clear your mind of noise.

Once you use it in your meditation and harness the energies of the unicorn merging it with yours, it is good to take with you when you need it. Keep it close to your heart and keep the energies flowing in the moments you need it the most.

Spirit Quartz

There are a few varieties of this sparkling stone like the amethyst, angel aura, and aqua aura. It can also be a clear stone but its defining feature is the tiny crystal points that make it twinkle.

The spirit quartz connects with unicorn energy to help strengthen family bonds, friendship bonds, inspires a person's creativity, and gives you an energy boost. It will help you harness the energy that fills a unicorn with wonder, love, inner peace, and joy.

Working with Crystals to Connect With a Unicorn's Energies and Light

Crystals should always be cleansed before using them for any purpose. They can be cleansed by running water or leaving them in the sunlight. You can even use both to ensure they are completely purified before aligning them with your purpose.

Take the crystal that you need and hold it in your right hand while you think of what you need to heal or gain. Feel it warm up in your palm as you open up the unicorn realm and align your intentions with the unicorn's consciousness.

Once you feel the warmth, power, and light carry the crystal with you. You can keep it in your pocket, wear it as a piece of jewelry, and place it beneath your pillow to sleep with at night.

You can also create a unicorn altar with a picture, statue, or symbol of a unicorn. Keep a nice perch upon which to place your crystal when you are not using it. The altar is also a good idea for meditation as you will be able to better draw in the unicorn with its image before you.

To use crystals during meditation, you need to take them with you when you transcend the light. Hold the desired crystal in your dominant hand and once you have opened your chakras and aligned the energy or ask the unicorn for help to heal what ails you. Use the gem to guide the unicorns light and energy to where you need it the most.

9

CHAPTER:
Sound Frequency and the Chakras

Each of the seven internal chakras has a unique corresponding frequency. Since each chakra vibrates at a unique frequency you can learn how to influence the frequency of the chakras to clear any blockages of energy and bring them into balance. Humans are alive with the frequencies of vibrations. Everything that makes you human– every cell, organ, emotion, feeling, and thought– all has its own unique frequency it vibrates at. When your chakras are open and spinning correctly your whole being is in harmony and balance. If the frequency of a chakra is out of balance then you will be out of balance, out of tune.

The key to healing your chakras with sound frequency is to find sounds on the same frequency as the chakra you are trying to heal and then spend time listening to it. The sounds are measured by the hertz unit (Hz), a unit of frequency of sound. It is the number of cycles, or vibrations, of the sound every second.

The Root Chakra frequency is 396 Hz. This measurement will free the energy of the Root Chakra and allow you to achieve your goals.

The Sacral Chakra frequency is 417 Hz, which will clear out the destructive energy and influences of the past events in your life. It will also open you to receiving a source of energy with no end, allowing you to completely change your life.

The Solar Plexus Chakra frequency is 528 Hz, which is the tone of the Sun. This frequency will bring great transformations into your life. It will also activate your intuition, intention, and imagination, allowing you to work toward your own highest purpose.

The Heart Chakra frequency is 639 Hz. This frequency will help you deal with relationship issues whether they are social in nature or problems with friends, partners, or family. This frequency will help your cells communicate with your environment.

The Throat Chakra frequency is 741 Hz, which will help you achieve a stable and pure life by leading you into the power of self-expression. This frequency is meant to cleanse and clear.

The Third Eye Chakra frequency is 852 Hz. The planet Venus is the same tone. This frequency will let you see through all of the illusions in your life. You will be able to see situations or people as they really are, not as they pretend to be. It will raise your personal awareness and help you get back to your spiritual order.

The Crown Chakra frequency is 963 Hz. This frequency enables direct experience and connects you with the light of the divine. With its help, you will be able to reconnect yourself with the spiritual higher world.

You can also help activate your chakras by chanting during meditation. When you are chanting the sounds inhale first and say the corresponding sound five times while you exhale. Each chakra has a sound which will mimic the frequency for that chakra:

Root Chakra – Lam, pronounced Lahm

Sacral Chakra – Vam, pronounced Vahm

Solar Plexus Chakra – Ram, pronounced Rahm

Heart Chakra – Yam, pronounced Yahm

Throat Chakra – Ham, pronounced Hahm

Third Eye Chakra – Ohm

Crown Chakra – Om

By listening to sounds at the proper frequencies and chanting the mantras for each chakra, you will soon become attuned to the finer frequencies your body emits until all of your chakras are spinning in the proper frequency.

10

CHAPTER:
Healing the Earth Star Chakra

Your Earth Star Chakra is located below your feet between one and three feet underground. This chakra helps you remain one with the earth you walk on. It holds the collective consciousness of all of humanity and is connected to the vastness of the Universe. When you activate, heal, and balance your Earth Star Chakra, you are also completing healing work for all of humanity and clearing the way for your connection with both all of humanity and the earth. This chakra is directly connected to all of the earth.

When you want to reach higher into the spiritual realms above you, you will need to make sure you are properly anchored into the earth with the help of the Earth Star Chakra. You will be balanced and clear in your daily life when this chakra is balanced and clear. You will have the ability to function in the reality of the physical world while you search to bring the vibrations and light of the higher realms of spirituality into a more physical form.

You can simply and easily activate this chakra by relaxing. It is best if you can relax outside in some sort of natural setting. If possible, lay down right in the grass, or at least on a lounge chair or in a hammock. If you can be near a source of running water, that is even better. Close your eyes, lie back, and relax. You will soon be filled with the vibrations of thankfulness and gratitude. Connect with the earth in your mind and allow this connection to help activate, balance, and cleanse your Earth Star Chakra.

Picture a bright white light streaming up from the very core of the earth and surrounding you with its soft warmth. Feel this light flowing through your body, through your centers of energy, and out the top of your head. See a beam of bright white light streaming down from above and meeting with the light from the earth. Feel these lights grounding you to the earth, grounding your energy, holding you safely as you reach for the stars. Feel your new oneness with the earth and all of existence.

Picture the light from the earth filling your Earth Star Chakra. Let yourself feel the healing restoration of this chakra. You need to activate the Earth Star Chakra if you want to be able to reach higher. It is the foundation for all of the other chakras, both internal and external. This is not a one-time activity, but something you will need to do every chance you get. Anytime you have the opportunity to get out into nature is another opportunity to reactivate this chakra.

As you allow yourself to be open to the full light and power of the Earth Star Chakra, you will feel it grow and build inside you. You will need to be fully in harmony with everything and everyone on earth if you want to fully activate your Earth Star Chakra. Learn to love all of life and nature and express gratitude for it as it surrounds you. Enjoy the peace and beauty of the sky, sun, moon, oceans, forests, mountains, and any part of nature out there. With the help of the earth you will keep your Earth Star Chakra healthy, and it will keep you well-grounded while you reach for the stars.

11

CHAPTER:
Healing the Root Chakra

Your Root Chakra is the foundation for your overall health and well-being. When this chakra is open and balanced you will feel prosperous, secure, relaxed, trusting, stable, and healthy. You will have plenty of energy as well as the ability to think clearly in all areas of your life. The characteristics of a balanced Root Chakra include feelings of calmness, centeredness, and being prepared for whatever life throws at you. You will be the person with unyielding common sense, and you will be physically and mentally at ease with yourself.

When your Root Chakra is not balanced, when it is closed or unhealthy, you can suffer from physical disorders of your bowels like diarrhea and constipation. You might also suffer from chronic illnesses, random body aches and pains, eating disorders, and anxiety. You might experience feelings of insecurity, paranoia, vulnerability, inability to relax, and aggression if there is an imbalance or blockage in this chakra. You might lack the confidence needed to achieve your goals or you may continuously struggle to succeed.

When you heal your Root Chakra, you will make a major impact on your life. There are many easy ways to do this.

As was already mentioned, red is the corresponding color of the Root Chakra. Imagine a pool of the color red covering the base of your spine. See this pool warming and protecting your Root Chakra. See this pool flowing down your legs and grounding you to the earth through your Earth Star Chakra. Surround yourself with the color red by wearing red clothing or putting out red accessories in your home.

Use essential oils with an earthy essence like frankincense, sandalwood, or patchouli. Burn some incense of these scents or put some essential oil in a fragrance diffuser.

The Root Chakra likes red foods and any root vegetables. Fill your kitchen with apples, cherries, carrots, beets, and onions. Surround your home and outdoor space with healing red or black stones like jet, smoky quartz, hematite, garnet, bloodstone, red jasper, or red carnelian.

Any kind of movement will help activate your Root Chakra. Dance to any kind of music you love. Do different yoga poses like tree pose, downward dog, Warrior I and II, and Mountain Pose. Go outside and go for a walk. Feel all of the energy you receive from the earth and nature. If you can walk around in your bare feet, that is even better. Do some work in your yard or plant a garden. Join events in your local community or get out and meet your neighbors.

Keep notes in a journal about any concerns you have about your Root Chakra. Write down the things that make you feel supported in your life, or what you need to help yourself feel supported. Think about how strong your personal roots are. Note any time you think things about yourself limiting you and your abilities. Write down any goals you want to achieve and note areas where you might need to be stronger.

When your Root Chakra is strong you will have a strong foundation for your own health and for the stability of your other chakras. Your confidence and energy will increase as your Root Chakra grows stronger. You will no longer be driven by fear and guilt. You will finally have the knowledge your life is going according to your plan and that everything will work out just fine.

12

CHAPTER:
Healing the Sacral Chakra

Your Sacral Chakra is the internal center of your sexual, emotional, and creative energy. If you pay attention to your actions, thoughts, feelings, and the physical sensations of your body, you will know when you need to cleanse and balance your Sacral Chakra. There are many signs indicating this chakra needs healing. You might have disorders of your stomach, kidneys, or lower back. You overthink everything or your creativity is stagnating. You might be emotionally aloof or extremely sensitive. You feed on others' drama. You have no energy and are always exhausted. You suffer from reproductive or sexual issues. You might either feel absolutely no emotion, or you might be overly emotional in any situation. You are addicted to feeling pleasure, and you find it wherever you can, in drink, food, drugs, gambling, work, compulsive shopping, or any other area you can find to do something to excess.

When your Sacral Chakra is healthy you will feel comfortable with yourself just the way you are. You will enjoy your sexuality and be able to enjoy it in balanced and healthy ways. Life will bring you pleasure without being excessive.

You will once again be emotionally grounded, and you will also be emotionally open. Your creativity will soar, and the small things in life will give you great pleasure once again. There are many ways to heal, cleanse, and balance your Sacral Chakra.

Take some time to explore your own creativity with activities that make you happy or look like they might be fun. Try something you have not done before. Look into activities like cooking, jewelry making, quilting, drawing, photography, sculpting, or sewing. Remember that some creative crafts take more time to learn than others, so be patient with yourself if you find something you really enjoy doing. Try to put your heart and soul into your new activities.

Think about the things you learned about sex and sexuality as a child and decide which ones no longer suit your lifestyle. The ideas you were taught are not the ideas you need to live with forever. These ideas might be exactly what is blocking your Sacral Chakra, so take the time to get to know yourself and the things that make you happy.

When you have holes in your life, you will try to fill them with whatever makes you happy at the moment. This is how addictions begin. Try to think about where your thoughts and feelings were when you became addicted to whatever addiction you might be fighting. Spend some time learning what it is you are trying to hide from or what you lack in your life. Also, take some time to think about your emotions and your emotional triggers. These may be the key to what drives your addictions.

Work with the color orange, the color corresponding with the Sacral Chakra. Surround yourself with this color. Wear one orange garment or piece of jewelry. Lay orange throws or soft cloths around your home. Eat more orange-colored food like oranges, carrots, apricots, mangos, sweet potatoes, papaya, and peaches. Even setting out a bowl of oranges, nectarines, or tangerines on your kitchen counter will help.

Embrace your body as it is now and stop hating the way you look. This is not to say you should not make changes if you are not happy with the way you look, but you need to accept yourself as you are first. Explore guided meditations for body affirmations. Experiment with different healthy foods and ways of eating. Cut out processed foods. Add grated ginger to hot dishes or drink ginger tea. Join an exercise class. Learn to do yoga, especially pigeon pose, reverse warrior, goddess, camel, butterfly, and cobra.

Meditate with guided meditations or daily affirmations. Use essential oils to clear out blockages in your Sacral Chakra. The best ones are bergamot, rosewood, jasmine, neroli, orange, and ginger. Chant out loud for the sound and vibration. Do something you normally would not do, something spontaneous. Go out to dinner alone. Watch a movie that normally would not interest you. Read a book in a different genre. Drive a different route to work.

Choose some or all of these activities and give them a try. Not all will be right for you, but you also might find a new interest you never knew you had. Decide exactly what kind of help your Sacral Chakra needs, and then work on it. Make notes of what works and what does not. Don't feel you need to stay with an activity if it is not working for you, but give all the activities you attempt a fair trial. Pay attention to the things making you feel good, and then do more of it.

13

CHAPTER:
Healing the Solar Plexus Chakra

B ecause your Solar Plexus Chakra will shine brightly like the sun when it is balanced, it is sometimes referred to as the lustrous gem of the energy centers in the body. When your Solar Plexus Chakra is harmonious, healthy, and functioning in its best possible state, you will feel self-confidence, self-control, and a great inner drive.

Unfortunately, many mindsets, habits, and traumatic experiences in your life can cause this chakra to become stagnant, suppressed, or blocked. If your parents were authoritarian figures, if you were bullied as a child, or if your upbringing was very strict, your Solar Plexus Chakra is most likely unhealthy or dysfunctional. This will also happen if you suffered from physical, emotional, sexual, or mental abuse at any time in your life, but especially as a child. And if your childhood was riddled with ideologies making you feel powerless– like social, traditional, or religious beliefs– then your Solar Plexus Chakra probably needs healing and balancing.

Since this chakra is the center of your self-esteem and your willpower, it is important for it to be functioning well. It is associated with the element of fire and is responsible for regulating all of your energy associated with your vitality, identity, intention, and action. You will know if your Solar Plexus Chakra needs healing by paying attention to your physical sensations, as well as your actions, feelings, and thoughts. If this chakra needs healing you probably carry excess weight around your middle and suffer from constipation, stomach upsets, or frequent gas. You might also have hypoglycemia, diabetes, ulcers, and irritable bowel syndrome. You will always be very hot or very cold, and you will usually feel lazy and fatigued. Most of your personal relationships will be co-dependent because you have trouble forming personal boundaries. You are either a person with low self-esteem who constantly seeks approval from others, or you have an overly inflated ego and like to dominate and bully other people. You are either powerless and weak or manipulative. You are probably addicted to one or more substances.

If your Solar Plexus Chakra is excessive, then you will be manic or aggressively energetic. If it is deficient, then you will be numb or passive. When too much energy flows in, the chakra is excessive and you will be aggressive, reactive, agitated, and overly lively. If not enough energy flows in, then the chakra is deficient and you will feel blocked, passive, sluggish, and lifeless.

When your Solar Plexus Chakra is harmonious, clear, and strong, you will be self-confident, comfortable in your own skin, and you will trust in your own abilities. Your constant struggles with aggressive egotism or self-doubt will be a thing of the past. You will understand you have the power to choose how you will feel and think and how you will approach other people and life in general. You will feel more self-assured, and you will possess the willpower and energy to make healthy boundaries taking care of you. You will be better able to stand your ground with more respect for others and yourself, so you will no longer have episodes of self-minimizing or explosive anger. The physical energy you find will drive you to move away from your addictive tendencies and your lethargy. You will once again drive yourself to achieve your dreams and goals. You will be aligned with life; empowered, focused, and energized.

Use essential oils to heal your Solar Plexus Chakra. Sandalwood, clove, cypress, rosemary, cinnamon, and black pepper work especially well. Wear a diffusing pendant as jewelry; put a few drops into an oil diffuser or wear a bit of diluted essential oil on your wrists. Certain crystals will help you to heal this chakra. Wear jewelry or carry the crystals with you. The best ones are yellow calcite, tiger's eye, citrine, topaz, and amber. Different herbs will help you to clear and ground the Solar Plexus Chakra. Use ginger, marshmallow leaf, lemongrass, rosemary, or chamomile in your cooking, or to make a great tasting tea. And certain foods will bring balance and health to this chakra. You will want to focus on eating more whole grains like rye, spelt, oats, and rice. Your diet should include a lot of legumes like beans, chickpeas, and lentils. Spices will help warm your body, so focus on using cinnamon, cumin, ginger, and turmeric when you cook. And yellow vegetable and fruits such as pineapple, corn, bananas, and lemons will help you to feel better almost immediately.

Try to keep your distance from people who are overly critical or like to bully you in any way. If you can't cut ties with them completely then try to limit your contact with them as much as possible. You will want to be with supportive people who will help build you up, not unsupportive people who will just drag you down. This is your power, and it is up to you to use it. You get to decide who leaves your life and who stays. And while you are cleaning up the excess people in your life try breaking out of your dull, safe routines and do something different every now and then. Even changing one or two people or small parts of your routine will give you a boost of vitality and energy and renew your energy levels.

And you will really need to spend some quiet time getting to know yourself and what it is you want out of life. You need to learn what it is you are constantly fighting against and what things fill you with fear. You will need to be honest with yourself so you can grow and develop. Usually people with an unhealthy or blocked Solar plexus Chakra will spend a lot of time suppressing or avoiding something or fighting against it. Get rid of any anger you are storing inside of you. Doing so is a great way to rapidly unblock your chakra. When you release the stored anger, you will have plenty of room for energy again.

Remember you are no longer the victim you were before. You are no longer defenseless and powerless. You also will no longer blame other people for your problems, and you will also not sacrifice your own needs to satisfy someone else's needs. Playing the victim takes too much of your precious energy. Try saying 'no' once in a while. Don't be rude or angry, but turn down suggestions or situations not appealing to you. Remember the victim does not need to take responsibility for them, and you are now taking control of your life. Try laughing at yourself every now and then. You will be surprised at how good it makes you feel.

Use positive affirmations for guided meditation whenever possible. Remember to say, 'I am,' 'I can,' and 'I will.' Begin each day with a few positive affirmations. Say them while you meditate or while you are firmly in your yoga poses. These techniques will bring about a feeling of positivity leaving no room for any negativity. Break free of unhealthy attachments by asking yourself why you are holding onto these outdated, useless ideas. If an object, memory, desire, or belief is not serving your highest good, get rid of it.

And one of the best ways to heal your Solar Plexus Chakra is to take care of yourself every day of your life. Your energy will become harmonious when you take care of your psychological and physical health. Stop neglecting your spiritual, mental, physical, and emotional health. Take better care of your body. Taking care of yourself is a form of self-love and self-respect. So set some goals for yourself and spend time working toward them. You will definitely be surprised at how much better you feel and how much more rewarding your life will be.

14

CHAPTER:
Healing the Heart Chakra

Your Heart Chakra is the center of your balance, love, and unity. When your Heart Chakra is healthy and open, you will feel generous, accepting, forgiving, receptive, open, and connected to other people and to yourself. If your Heart Chakra is unhealthy or blocked, you will feel fear, bitterness, resentment, loneliness, and social isolation. This chakra can suffer due to many different factors. If you were raised by a parent who was a narcissist or was cold and unfeeling then your Heart Chakra likely needs healing. If you were denied love and affection while you were growing up or you suffered from emotional or physical abuse, then this chakra will need healing. The Heart Chakra will be blocked from receiving and giving love if you have self-destructive habits or harbor unhealthy beliefs about love and affection.

As the center of your balance, love, and connection with other people, the Heart Chakra is responsible for regulating the energy inside of you associated with openness, compassion, self-love, self-acceptance, and your unconditional love for other people. When you heal this chakra you will support, cleanse, clear, and open it to giving and receiving love. Physically, people with an unhealthy Heart Chakra will feel a tightness or heaviness in their chests and might develop problems in the chest, lungs, or heart such as poor circulation, high blood pressure, and asthma. You mistrust other people and are suspicious of their motives toward you. Your relationships are built on co-dependency and you struggle to freely give and receive love. You might be excessively fearful, self-critical, anxious, or needy. The trauma you have suffered is constantly replaying in your heart and mind. You are critical of yourself and jealous of others. You might hold grudges and find it difficult to let go of your angry and bitter thoughts and feelings. You swing between being terrified of being alone and being distant emotionally in your relationships.

A deficient Heart Chakra will cause you to feel self-critical, isolated, and anxious. An overly expressive Heart Chakra will make you feel clingy, prone to smothering displays of affection and love, and easily adopt the role of a martyr. When your Heart Chakra is harmonious, clear, and strong, you will feel receptive and open. You will have the courage to open your heart to other people and you will no longer feel bitterness, fear, and isolation. You will know the best way to receive love is to be able to give love to others. Your relationship with yourself will be built on self-love and self-acceptance. And even when others try to hurt you, your heart will remain soft and open.

You will be able to release all of the old, toxic ideas about love that used to define your relationships. You will trust your instincts more and will easily give up the role of martyr or victim. You will be able to express more understanding and compassion when you are better able to love and trust yourself. In time you will feel more forgiving, receptive, expansive, and loving. There are many easy ways to balance and heal your Heart Chakra.

Since green is the color of the Heart Chakra, start spending more time in nature. Get outside to any place lush with greenery. If you live in the city, try growing a small garden or fill your home with house plants.

When your heart is balanced, it is beautiful and shares its loving kindness with others freely. Try a little loving meditation to heal your Heart Chakra. And do not be afraid to set personal boundaries. If you often use the word 'yes' when you would rather say 'no,' you need to take inventory of your priorities and set some personal limits. If you are desperately trying to make everyone else happy, there is no way you will ever make yourself happy. Take better care of yourself and your heart by learning to be gently assertive.

Herbs like angelica, hops, nettle, hawthorn, holy basil, astragalus, and rose are best for clearing and opening the Heart Chakra. Drinking them as a soothing tea is the best method. Certain energetic crystals will help you to heal your Heart Chakra. Carry or meditate with chrysocolla, green fluorite, ruby, prehnite, rhodonite, emerald, rose quartz, malachite, and jade. Certain essential oils like angelica, neroli, lavender, ylang-ylang, rose, and marjoram will heal this chakra. Adding green foods to the diet will greatly enhance the health of your Heart Chakra. Try celery, grapes, zucchini, peppers, cabbage, avocados, peas, broccoli, lettuce, chard, pears, green apples, kale, spinach, and kiwis. And try different yoga poses for cleansing, especially fish pose, camel, eagle, cat, cobra, and forward bend.

When your mind is overly judgmental, it will be difficult to show love for others. Learn to clear these thoughts from your mind. Do not take personally the slights other people send your way, but try to think of what they might be feeling at that time. Give yourself permission to feel love for yourself and others. Your emotions are meant to be embraced and used, not shut out, repressed, or controlled. Allow yourself to be jealous, bored, sad, angry, or unhappy as you need to be.

Become accustomed to the feeling of a hug. Learn to hug others and let them hug you. And let yourself receive love from others. Do not push away the love that others want to show you. Don't deny compliments or affection, but receive them graciously.

Don't take life and love for granted, but practice counting your blessings. Acknowledge all of the good things you have in your life, and try to let go of all of the dark energy your mind and body are storing. This is the place where you store all of your denied and rejected habits, feelings, thoughts, personality traits, and unacceptable ego. When you loosen these areas and begin to release them, your heart will open a bit more with every release.

Forgive yourself. Think of all the ways and all the times when you mistreated yourself or did not take good care of yourself. Let go of any resentment or anger you might be holding toward someone else. Stop playing the role of victim or martyr. These roles are driven by low self-esteem, which has no place in the person with a healthy Heart Chakra. Try on different roles such as helper, peacemaker, confidant, or friend. Do one nice thing for yourself and for someone else every day. Try to be a thoughtful person. Use affirmations for guided meditation if that helps you to become more loving, like those suggested in Chapter 6. And don't forget to laugh as often as you possibly can. Laughter is one of the best healers we have available.

15

CHAPTER:
Healing the Throat Chakra

When your Throat Chakra is balanced and healthy, you will be assertive, confidant, honest, creative, and not afraid of expressing your truth. If your Throat Chakra is blocked you will struggle with problems such as verbal aggressiveness, lack of creativity, untrustworthiness, stubbornness, dishonesty, social anxiety, shyness, and a fear of expressing your thoughts. If you feel like your Throat Chakra is unhealthy or blocked think about your life as a child. If you were not able to express your real thoughts and feelings, if your opinions were not important, if you were often criticized by authority figures, then your Throat Chakra might need cleansing and balancing. Your Throat Chakra is the chakra responsible for regulating the energy inside of you associated with understanding, creativity, and authenticity.

You will know when your Throat Chakra is closed, blocked, or unhealthy. Physically you will regularly develop upper respiratory infections, throat infections, or sinus infections. You might have ear infections or premature hearing loss.

Your lymph nodes might be swollen, your voice might sound thin, nasally, or crack a lot, or you may have hypothyroidism or hyperthyroidism. You will find it hard to be honest with others and yourself, and you might do one thing but say another thing. In your relationships you are the quiet one, allowing your partner to make all of the decisions. The idea of public speaking paralyzes you, and you have trouble finding your own voice among others. You are either highly over-opinionated or painfully shy in a crowd. Conversations make you feel anxious. You will either force your personal beliefs on other people or you will struggle nervously when you try to share your own opinions. A fear of being accepted by others causes you to keep your feelings and thoughts secret because you often feel misunderstood or ignored by other people. Miscommunication is no stranger to you.

If your Throat Chakra is excessively open you will communicate with anger, hold on to your stubborn ideas, and tend to be overbearing socially. If your Throat Chakra is deficient you will live in secrecy, suffer from shyness, and have problems expressing your thoughts and feelings. When this chakra is harmonious, clear, and strong, you will be honest, open, fluent, and not afraid to let others know how you really feel. Your ability to confidently express your feelings and thoughts will be amazing. You will share your truths freely no matter what happens or what other people think. Use the following methods to open, balance, and heal your Throat Chakra.

Use the affirmations provided in Chapter 6 as guided meditation to heal this chakra. Use humming mantras or sound therapy, since the Throat Chakra is especially receptive to both of these. Keep a private journal of your deepest thoughts and feelings. Make it a point to write something in your journal every day so you can get into the habit of expressing your feelings. Don't pay any attention to your grammar or your sentence structure while you are writing, but let your feelings flow freely.

The corresponding color of the Throat Chakra is blue, so add into your diet blue foods such as grapes, blackberries, blueberries, currants, and plums. Some foods resonating with this chakra are apricots, figs, peaches, pears, lemons, grapefruit, apples, and kiwis. Slippery elm, clove, fennel, echinacea, spearmint, cinnamon, and elderberry are some of the herbs that help heal the Throat Chakra. They are best used for making a soothing tea. Since this chakra loves the color blue so much, surround yourself with it. Stare up at the sky or out at a body of blue water. Wear blue clothing, and toss blue blankets and pillows around your furniture. Crystal energy can be found with lapis lazuli, aquamarine, azurite, tanzanite, larimar, and blue kyanite. Yoga poses helpful for healing this chakra are plow pose, lion pose, and fish pose. And surround yourself with the scents of essential oils like myrrh, rosemary, clove, eucalyptus, neroli, ylang-ylang, and frankincense. Always try to drink pure water.

Ground yourself by practicing deep breathing. When your Throat Chakra is unbalanced, you will tend to speak impulsively or too quickly. Calm yourself with deep breaths helping to center and ground you. While you are practicing your breathing silently give thanks to life and to the universe for supporting your life. Learn to listen to other people when they are speaking. When this chakra has too much energy, you will try to dominate conversations. Deep breathing will also help you break this habit. Breathe slowly and deeply while you focus on listening to other people and the words they are saying.

Singing, screaming, and laughing are all good ways to release excess built-up energy stuck in your throat. Laughing or screaming allows you to let go of frustrations and negativity. And singing is probably the most beautiful and natural way to open your Throat Chakra. You do not need to sing in front of other people if you are self-conscious. Sing in the car with the windows rolled up tightly. Turn the radio volume up and enjoy yourself.

Silence is also a good way to heal this chakra. It lets you tune up your subtle inner voice. This will allow it to emerge and make itself known to you. A soothing neck massage is always a good idea for relaxing this chakra. And if you are not comfortable with being assertive, you could practice when you are alone.

16

CHAPTER:
Healing the Third Eye Chakra

The energy center in your body responsible for your intuition, thought, manifesting, perception, and reality is your Third Eye Chakra. When this chakra is opened, a doorway to spiritual enlightenment is opened. When this chakra is balanced and clean, you will possess emotional balance, self-awareness, insight, strong intuition, and clarity. If the Third Eye Chakra is closed or unhealthy, you will struggle with mood disorders, mental illnesses, paranoia, depression, anxiety, cynicism, and closed-mindedness. This chakra can easily become damaged in childhood if you were raised in a family of close-minded people who taught you to be obedient and never question authority.

When this chakra is unhealthy, closed, or blocked, you will physically suffer from migraines, sinus problems, vision problems, and earaches. You will either be ungrounded and dreamy or opinionated and arrogant. You will be stubborn and find it difficult to be open-minded. You will find it difficult to like other people. Your relationships and interactions with others will be superficial or trivial because you will easily dislike or mistrust others. Your opinions of the world will be rigid and nearly impossible to change. Reality will not be clear to you and you will have problems connecting to your soul or your deeper self. You might also be addicted to things making you feel pleasure like status, money, sex, shopping, drink, food, or relationships.

A balanced and open Third Eye Chakra will make it easier for you to be more objective in your opinions and less rigid in your beliefs. Your life will be more fluid and free-flowing, and this will allow you to be more spontaneous and creative. You will feel more compassion and wisdom, and this will let you reach your mystical state of being much easier. This chakra might be a bit more difficult to heal since it involves a lot of soul growth.

It is important to explore new points of view if you truly want to heal this chakra. This will assist you in breaking the cycle of being close-minded and rigid in your beliefs. You will also be easily lost in delusion and fantasy if you are not grounded in reality. Try to work on being present in your everyday life, and do not allow your mind to wander off too far.

Get outside and enjoy some sunlight every day. This will help to heal the Third Eye Chakra because it will help clear your mind. Use blue lotus, rosemary, passionflower, lavender, jasmine, basil, saffron, star anise, or mugwort herbs in cooking or as incense. These will also make delicious teas. Add into your diet more of the purple foods the Third Eye Chakra enjoy like purple potatoes, purple carrots, purple kale, purple cabbage, eggplant, raisins, figs, blueberries, blackberries, dates, and prunes. Use Third Eye Chakra appropriate essential oils like vetiver, juniper, sandalwood, clary sage, frankincense, and patchouli. Amethyst, labradorite, kyanite, lapis lazuli, sapphire, and shungite crystal can be carried or worn. Work on your yoga poses, especially head-to-knee poses, child's pose, dolphin pose, and standing forward bend. Light a candle and set it three to four feet in front of you and stare at the flame. Keep your vision focused in an easy, natural way.

One of the reasons this chakra will be damaged is when you hold on to limiting core beliefs. Your core beliefs are the deep convictions you hold true that make you feel self-loathing, insecurity, and fear. When you are able to uncover those core beliefs you keep hidden, you will be able to open this chakra and keep it healthy. Try to be more self-aware, as this is a necessary skill you need to develop. It will help you increase your self-awareness. Keep a private journal of your deepest feelings and thoughts. Go outside at night and stare at the moon, especially if it is full.

The main reason the Third Eye Chakra becomes unhealthy or blocked is because you identify with the thoughts you are thinking because you believe in them. Learn how to observe your thoughts without thinking they are the ultimate truth. Feelings and thoughts do not have any meaning unless we give them a meaning. And keep in mind your dreams express your inner needs, fears, and desires. They are naturally rich in symbols holding meaning for your life. You interpret your dreams with the help of your Third Eye Chakra.

And always remember to tell yourself how well you are doing. Use positive affirmations as guided meditation to heal and balance your Third Eye Chakra. Use phrases beginning with the words 'I see,' 'I trust,' or 'I create,' as further outlined in Chapter 6.

17

CHAPTER:
Healing the Crown Chakra

The highest of the internal chakras is the Crown Chakra. It is the energy center of your consciousness on a cosmic level. The Crown Chakra connects you to the eternal because it is the seat of your divine awareness. You easily connect to your higher self when this chakra is balanced and open. You feel a sense of wholeness and serenity, easily see the big picture, feel connected to life and other people, and tap into your inner wisdom. Living in environments full of unresolved stress and trauma can lead to your Crown Chakra being blocked or unhealthy.

When this chakra is blocked or unhealthy, you will suffer from endocrine and neurological disorders. You might have migraines or be sensitive to bright light. You may have mental illnesses that involve delusions. You will suffer from chronic fatigue, mental confusion and fog, insomnia, nightmares, or night terrors. You will be lonely, greedy, materialistic, and disconnected spiritually. Your sense of self will be limited and very rigid. You will think narrow minded thoughts and keep yourself isolated from other people. Your ego might be out of control because you lack any feelings of compassion and care toward other people.

Your Crown Chakra is your access to enlightenment and the window to your soul. Crown Chakra healing will make you feel more enlightened as well as giving you more clarity and inner peace. Your former sense of isolation will be replaced by a feeling of being connected with all of humanity. You will belong. Your perspective will be rejuvenated, and you will no longer feel bored with life. Living will once again be beautiful. You will feel more playful, light, and fluid as you become less rigid and begin to lose your ego. You will live more in the moment and better see the big picture of life. Your reality will be defined by serenity and expansiveness.

One of the easiest and most important ways to heal and balance your Crown Chakra is by meditation. Use your affirmations as guided meditations. Do not become too immersed in your own thoughts, but try to let them flow freely. Find a quiet place to relax and turn your attention inside yourself. See the thoughts floating around in your mind. Think of how they arrived without even thinking of them. Your thoughts arise spontaneously so there is no reason for you to think your thoughts should define you.

Break out of your comfort zone and your limiting thoughts by reading books or watching movies you normally would not enjoy. Work to identify those areas of prejudice or ignorance you need to work on. As you spend more time reading and hearing the thoughts of others, you will have less time to dwell on your limiting thoughts.

Declutter your life by simplifying your surroundings. Emotional and mental distress are caused and aggravated by an excess of mess and belongings. When you simplify and clean your environment you will also be purifying yourself. By cleaning the external environment, you make it easier to clean the internal environment. When you have made space available by removing the things you don't need or want, you will have room to create a space for your own daily spiritual practice. Make a small area designated as the place you will go to get in touch with your spiritual self. Put things meaning something to you there, like incense, crystals, candles, books, or stones. Take things from around your house meaningful to you and put them in your special place. The way you conduct your spiritual practice will be unique to you. You might do rituals, pray, practice yoga, sing, meditate, read, study, or simply be. Also take some time each day to pray. This does not necessarily mean praying to God or to only say religious prayers. You can pray to whatever being you feel most drawn to, like the Soul, Spirit, Ancestors, Goddess or God, Life, or Spirit Guides. Prayer is very beneficial and very simple.

Look for communication from the Spirit and signs that he is speaking to you. You will need to be open to the guidance happening all around you. If you are feeling cynical you will cut the ties between your surroundings and your mind, body, and soul. Be brave enough to question the beliefs you have held all your life and see if you need to make changes. Cynicism usually comes from a sense of worthlessness and insecurity. Work to overcome your low sense of self-esteem.

Don't forget your affirmations for guided meditation. Always use phrases that begin with the words 'I am,' 'I see,' and 'I trust.' For more detailed affirmation examples, refer back to Chapter 6.

18

CHAPTER:
Healing the Causal Chakra

The purpose of your Causal Chakra is to accept energy from your Soul Star Chakra and filter it into your aura. This chakra deals with higher wisdom and the exploration of your spirit. It opens when your right brain is activated, and it will help you to see the big picture using creativity and intuition. Through this chakra you will receive messages, inspiration, and information from the higher spiritual realms. To be able to do this you will need to separate yourself from the beliefs you have probably held onto all your life, beliefs holding you back from achieving true enlightenment. When information is received through the Causal Chakra, it is filtered down through all of the other chakras.

Before you can activate this chakra, it will need to be responsive, open, and free from any belief systems you might have programmed into it. If this chakra is out of balance or overloaded, you will not be able to get rid of the memories of old experiences, behaviors, and patterns. You will continue to gather similar experiences into your life, and you will get stuck in an endless cycle of regret, guilt, and self-judgment. When you activate this chakra, you will alter your perceptions, and you will broaden all the horizons of your consciousness. Your inferior mental programs and patterns will be flooded with spiritual meaning. This will let you remain peaceful and calm even when your life is full of trials.

When the Causal Chakra is first activated it is not attached to the head but is located next to it, between the Crown Chakra and the Soul Star Chakra. As the level of light inside rises, it will move closer to you so that it is very near your Crown Chakra. This chakra is directly connected to the healing energy of the moon and its healing powers. It absorbs and radiates a divine feminine light. This chakra pulls light from the heavens down into you and your centers of energy. This will illuminate the deep wisdom you hold in your soul and will also raise your vibrations.

The divine feminine is known as one of the most powerful energies that has come to earth recently. The moon plays a large part in the spreading of this energy, since it also holds feminine energy and helps dispense it to us. The moon also reflects the light from the sun, which gives us energy and warmth. During periods of full moon humanity is flooded with the powerful silver light radiating from the moon.

Sensitive people and animals will be affected profoundly by the vibrations emitted by the moon and by the full moon itself. The Causal Chakra also has another amazing purpose in your life; it will give you an intimate and deep connection to the Spirit world. The psychic gifts you brought from your past life will determine how connected you will be to the spirit world through your Causal Chakra. When the light comes through the Causal Chakra and illuminates your Crown Chakra, the unicorns will assist in lighting up your energy fields. This light has the ability to completely alter the path of your soul.

19

CHAPTER:
Healing the Soul Star Chakra

If you have ever experienced intuitive nudges or flashes of memory about your past lives, you may have already connected with your Soul Star Chakra. Your Soul Star Chakra is the seat of your soul, even though it's found above your head. The name comes from your direct connection to your karmic past, your higher self, and your past lives. This chakra is where your soul stores its memories. It carries all the information pertaining to your purpose for being here and the information about your soul's past. You would not naturally know this information; only by activating the Soul Star Chakra will you have access to it.

When you activate this chakra, you will have a powerful tool for activating the remainder of your chakras. This chakra is directly connected to your higher self and to the light coming from the universe. This is a powerful energy that can be used to keep your Crown Chakra healthy and open. The Soul Star Chakra is the key to all of the information about your past lives and your karmic past. The chakra is your direct link to all of this information. When you take the time to tap into the past lives you lived, you will be better able to understand your current life and your place in the universe. Another important benefit is the ability to understand the people and relationships in your current life.

There are several methods for activating and connecting with your Soul Star Chakra. One of the easiest is using crystals. Hold any crystals you want to use in your hands while you meditate. Lithium quartz will help you calm yourself on your journey. Clear quartz will help balance and heal the chakra. Selenite is a super cleansing crystal that will help you activate the Soul Star Chakra. Phenacite is a less common crystal, but very powerful when used for connecting with this chakra. And kyanite will gently balance and cleanse the Soul Star Chakra.

Try to have some level of curiosity when you begin the journey toward activating your Soul Star Chakra. Sit comfortably in a quiet place and hold your crystals if you have them. Focus on breathing deeply and slowly while you relax. Picture a bright white light over your head shining down on you. Picture this light focusing its strength on your Soul Star Chakra. The chakra is growing brighter and warmer. Ask the powers of the universe to help you activate your Soul Star Chakra. Repeat a verse or mantra if you like while you meditate. Something like 'I feel love' or 'I feel divine light' would be appropriate. As soon as you feel connected to your Soul Star Chakra, imagine the bright white light expanding to shine over all of your body and flow through all of your chakras, helping to balance and heal them. Close your meditation by letting the light fade and disappear back into the universe.

20

CHAPTER:
Healing the Universal Chakra

This chakra is located above your head and is a multi-faceted orb known as the Chakra of Universal Consciousness, or the Universal Chakra. This chakra will allow you to reach above the everyday world to reach a state of enlightenment and commune with the divine. This will let you stretch beyond your common realm of understanding to work into a sense of universal unity with all that exists. This chakra is the chakra of mastery of your soul's purpose through your human existence.

The Universal Chakra vibrates like a swirling sun full of color that can only be truly appreciated with the inner eye of the mind. This chakra is a reflection of the sun, and it burns brightly and is hot because the sun provides light, warmth, and energy. It is your source of power and strength and your ability to create change not only in the nonphysical dimension but the physical dimension as well.

Proper balancing and clearing of this chakra is necessary because it shows you have a healthy fear of leaving this earth. The energies of the universe and the ascension are a natural part of you, and you will have a sense something in your life is changing. You may be afraid of these changes and start blocking the energies from the chakra. Realize these energies will not carry you off the planet. This is the beginning of the process that can take many years to complete. It can happen at any time. You will not leave until you are completely ready and have finished what you came to do on Earth.

Activating this chakra will bring you to a level of knowledge and acceptance you have never before known. This chakra will bring you extra-sensory perception, cosmic wisdom, and divine knowledge. You will be able to see far beyond your body and your mind. You will be able to experience your existence in its purest form, and you will become completely aware of your place in the universe.

21

CHAPTER:
Healing the Divine Gateway Chakra

The Divine Gateway Chakra is a portal through which bright light can enter your consciousness. This light from the universe will help awaken all of the wisdom in your soul. The gateway is an important spiritual portal through which all the wisdom of the universe will come to you. You will use deep meditation to activate this chakra so that you can use it for your own greater good.

Sit somewhere comfortable in a place where you will not be disturbed for as long as you need to be there. Breathe in deeply and slowly, allowing your breath to leave just as slowly as it came in. Always fill your abdomen with each breath in order to awaken all of the internal chakras. Move your energy through your body with ten deep breaths.

On the last exhale shift your focus up, and this time let your breath flow up through the Divine Gateway. The next time you inhale it will come from the Divine Gateway Chakra. Let this breath flow down inside of you to circulate through all the energy centers inside of you. When you exhale send out any unwanted or extra energy your breath collected while circulating through your body. After four inhales and exhales begin to picture a light flowing from the universe down through the Divine Gateway Chakra.

Pause for just a moment and put your focus on your breathing. Also focus on the white light shining down upon you. Let the light expand until it is covering all of you with its soft warmth. Now that you have activated the Divine Gateway Chakra, it is time for you to travel back to a time before you came into this life, to a time when you travelled a different path in a different life. Picture in your mind what that life was like. See yourself back in that life as you reconnect with the feeling of being in that past time.

Breathe deeply in and bring with your breath the peace from that place where you once were. Let it become one with your soul; let it become part of your being. Continue breathing in and out, slowly and deeply, while you enjoy the peace of that past time mixing with the peace of now in the glow of the bright white light.

22

CHAPTER:
Healthy Chakras Healing Ailments

Some of the information about the chakras can be confusing, but it is all very easy to learn and understand. The most important consideration to remember is the overall effect your chakras will have on your health and well-being. Illnesses are caused in your body not just by bad luck in matters of health or by possessing bad genetics. You do not become sick just because you eat bad foods or by having bad habits. Spiritual and mental health plays a large part in how healthy you will feel as you go through your life.

Your outlook on your life, thoughts, and feelings you keep hidden in the darkest recesses of your mind all play a part in how healthy you will be during your life. The way you think and the words you use will also play a part in your health. Everything you do, think, or say will have something to do with your health. Your chakras hold all of the energy for your body and its functions. These centers of energy work together with your consciousness to control your connections to the physical and spiritual worlds.

As mentioned in the beginning, the energy flowing freely through your body is known as your 'chi,' and it enters your body through your Crown Chakra, coming directly from the divine power of the universe. It moves down your body from the top of your head as it disperses energy throughout your other chakras. As the energy travels downward through your body and your energy centers, it removes your negative energy and cleanses your negative emotions. When this ball of energy reaches the bottom of your Root Chakra, found at the end of your spinal column, it then turns and travels back up through your body and your chakras back to your Crown Chakra, where it is released back to the Higher Power.

Energy will not flow properly through your chakras if even just one of them is too open or too closed, since energy cannot flow freely through the chakras when that happens. When this happens, your soul will never be able to grow in maturity and understanding until all of your issues causing imbalanced and unhealthy chakras have been solved. The very balance of your body is reflected in the health of your chakras. Your body is a contained system where all your individual parts need to work together for the good of the system as a whole. If one of your organs or one of your chakras is not healthy or not balanced, then it will not perform to the best of its ability, and over time the integrity of the remainder of your body will be affected, causing diseases and illnesses. Your diseases and illnesses will be a direct result of your unbalanced and unhealthy chakras.

Your Root Chakra is aligned with the bundle of nerves that supply feeling to your abdomen and the buttocks. It controls your adrenal glands. It also controls the temperature of your body, the production of your blood, your spine, and your muscular and skeletal systems, and it has influence over the health of your kidneys. If your Root Chakra is not working properly it can cause slow wound healing, growth problems, allergies, leukemia and other cancers, blood disorders, ailments of the spine, and arthritis. If this chakra is open too far, you might experience the feelings of being isolated or alone in the world, and this may drive, you to seek out material possessions or to engage in loveless or selfish behavior.

ROOT CHAKRA – When your Root Chakra is in balance and opened you will feel more mentally and physically stable and secure. You will find it much easier to face your doubts and fears head-on because there will be a secure sense of stability making it easier for you to remain grounded while reaching high to achieve your dreams and goals. Stressful situations will not cause such a strong reaction as before because your body will fill itself with a sense of peace and calm. Stressful feelings will still occur, but the openness of the Root Chakra will make it so much easier to handle stressful situations peacefully. Your enthusiasm will be high, and especially the enthusiasm leading to fun in all areas of life, particularly with that special partner. Since the Root Chakra is the lowest chakra in the body it deals with primal instincts, and this includes all sexual instincts. By opening and balancing the Root Chakra a person will feel an amazingly overwhelming feeling of confidence, motivation, and courage. These feelings will replace doubts, fears, and anxieties and will allow living a life full of fun and pleasure.

In order to lead a happy and well-balanced life it is necessary to meet the needs of basic human survival. The overall security you feel in your daily life is greatly impacted by having money, food, and shelter. This is the reason why the Root Chakra is also known as the foundation of life and of the other chakras, and why it is settled at the end of the spine. When this Root Chakra is well-balanced it gives you a feeling of being anchored in reality and surrounded by calmness and security. When it is out of balance you will feel threatened, lost, panicky, and anxious.

SACRAL CHAKRA – Your Sacral Chakra is located near your pubic area and is responsible for the health of the testes, bladder, uterus, rectum, anus, large intestine, blood pressure, adrenal glands, testicles, prostate glands, kidneys, and ovaries. When this chakra is out of its regular healthy state it may cause sexual malfunction. It might also cause the following issues: menstrual irregularities, uterine problems, prostate problems, constipation, bladder ailments, kidney disease, problems with the lower back, and high blood pressure. Imbalances might also lead to extreme feelings of guilt, particularly in sexual matters, which can lead you to feeling severely emotionally drained. If your Sacral Chakra is strong, you are able to take care of yourself easily while still exhibiting empathy and understanding for other people. If the chakra closes completely, you will feel disconnected from the outside world. You will become reclusive, withdrawing from friends, family, and the company of others. You may also be unable to focus on yourself, and you will work tirelessly to help other people while neglecting yourself. If your chakra is too far open, you might have feelings of jealousy, manipulation, violence, and addictive behaviors.

When your Sacral Chakra is balanced and open it will be so much easier for you to discover creative solutions to old problems or to envision new ideas that weren't easily recognizable before. The creative side of your psyche will be open and aware. Making decisions will now be easier because your brain will no longer be operating at one level of thought but should be able to access all levels. Judgments should become clearer, which will then lead to better quality decision making. Your life will once again be filled with joy, in the simplicity of life and gain a renewed passion for life itself. By looking at life through a new view, thoughts and feelings not evident before will rise to the top of your consciousness. Inner peace will be a way of life. The ability to express feelings and thoughts without becoming emotionally attached to them will be the new standard. And it will be possible to tap into the consciousness of the universe to truly realize your formerly hidden potential.

Since your Sacral Chakra is located below your belly button near your pelvic region it is responsible for sexuality as well as creativity and emotional responses. An out of balance Sacral Chakra may lead to feelings of sexual shame or guilt, a lack of personal boundaries, difficulty empathizing with other people, and a surge of other emotional issues. A healthier attitude toward relationships and a marked boost in reproductive and artistic creativity should come with a balanced Sacral Chakra.

SOLAR PLEXUS CHAKRA – Your Solar Plexus Chakra is found in your stomach just above your belly button and just below your ribs. This chakra is responsible for your pancreas, spleen, diaphragm, gall bladder, liver, intestines, and stomach. If this chakra is unhealthy you can experience emotions like cruelty, violence, envy, hatred, greed, jealousy, and anger. When it is out of balance your desire to do better things in your life can accelerate into undesirable feelings of aggressiveness, high ambitions, a craving for fame and fortune, and an overdeveloped ego. The physical symptoms it can cause are asthma, high blood pressure, heart problems, and allergies of the skin, colitis, diabetes, hepatitis, diarrhea, constipation, ulcers, and digestive disorders. When your Solar Plexus Chakra is unbalanced or unhealthy it can bring feelings of shame and can cause you to question your own self-worth. This reflects in your body by causing your digestive processes to slow down. It can also cause you to have a negative attitude toward food and use it for comfort instead of for nutrition. If this chakra is open too wide you can experience low self-worth and self-esteem, poor motivation, a lack of confidence, and a lot of anger.

You will feel many benefits when you gain balance and openness in your Solar Plexus Chakra. When you open the power of this chakra it will give you greater personal power to gain control over your thoughts and emotions. You will be able to control reactions to the stresses of life and your own mental and emotional states. You will then have a huge advantage over your old ways of thinking because of the ability to stop worrying and stressing over inconsequential matters and the ability to think and feel in more positive ways.

Procrastination is something you will leave in the past. Unblocking this chakra will allow for your willpower and your personal energy to tackle projects immediately, even those ignored for a long time because of lack of interest. Inner energy will flow in great quantities through you to enable you to take direct action. This renewed level of energy will also allow for an opening of your thoughts and feelings that will flow from your open mind. Old beliefs limiting your progress will be left behind and unique out-of-the-box thinking will be enabled. Your enhanced level of spirituality will lead you to a greater sense of the inner workings of your mind and new insights into your deepest thoughts and feelings. Action and will power are governed by your Solar Plexus Chakra. Commitments and personal power radiate from this chakra. Having this chakra in balance will give you the strength that you need for inspiration and inner balance and it will aid you in letting go of unhealthy attachments and bad habits. Negative emotions like shame, despair, anger, and greed are manufactured by an unbalanced Solar Plexus Chakra.

HEART CHAKRA – Responsible for governing the circulatory system, heart, and lungs, your Heart Chakra is located in the very center of your chest. When it is kept well-balanced you will enjoy feelings of love, compassion, and empathy. When this chakra is not healthy it can create physical problems in your heart and lungs including tuberculosis, asthma, and bronchitis. If your Heart Chakra is blocked, you will feel a lot of grief and sadness. You may become overly concerned with your comfort and emotional security, and you might have problems displaying compassion and feelings self-acceptance. This chakra is powered by love, not just for other people but for self and all of the beings of the universe. The Heart Chakra wants to receive and give love freely and unconditionally.

Feeling empathy for other people is beneficial in all areas of your life, from work to home. Feeling and showing empathy for others also allows you a greater ability to relate to other people and to understand them better. You will enjoy a new sense of direction in your personal life, and unblocking the Heart Chakra will re-ignite the passion lying dormant inside of you. Once your heart is open love will flow freely from you to other people and from other people to you. Enhanced spiritual growth will lead to an overall wholeness of being, due to the exploration of your feelings and thoughts buried out of fear of their possibilities and outcomes.

Your Heart Chakra is the internal center for your compassion and love. Your life will be filled with love, forgiveness, acceptance, compassion, and kindness when this Chakra is open and balanced. Doubts, worries, and fears will be removed. The Heart Chakra gives off certain signs when it is out of balance, such as a feeling of unworthiness or being stuck in one place in life. It can also make you have an absorbing fear of rejection, harbor self-defeating thoughts and feelings, and neglect your own health and well-being in order to give more to other people. When completely open and balanced, you will once again be able to feel deep love for yourself and other people. It is necessary to feel love for yourself first before it is possible to feel deep love for others. By cleansing yourself of the negative thoughts and feelings leading to self-judgment, it will be possible to once again feel unconditional love for other people.

THROAT CHAKRA – The chakra responsible for your neck, mouth, tongue, hands, arms, lymphatic system, parathyroid, thyroid, trachea, voice box, and throat is your Throat Chakra. This chakra is also in charge of your emotions and feelings of aesthetics, speech, expression, creativity, and communicating. If the Throat Chakra is not kept healthy or is out of balance, then illness will develop such as tonsillitis and sore throats. This can also cause problems with your cervical spine, voice, and your thyroid gland. The negative emotions a blocked or unhealthy Throat Chakra can display include lying, deceit and a lack of personal integrity. This is because your voice is blocked from true honest speech, so your negative emotions are allowed to take over. If the chakra is open too widely, you will soon stop listening to the good advice other people have to offer. You will also be unable to listen to, or accept the opinions, of other people, or you might become extremely prejudiced.

The Throat Chakra, when balanced and opened, will give a new meaning to clear thinking. You will easily be able to make decisions that were pushed aside because of difficulty. You will soon find it is much easier for you to gain new friends and to achieve the goal of climbing the corporate ladder. Your thoughts and communications will flow forth effectively and clearly. Balancing the Throat Chakra will enable you to speak freely with words of truth, love, and kindness. It will give you the ability to enlighten and inspire other people with your words because you will always choose the right ones. When you find yourself struggling to find the right words, avoid speaking the plain truth. Similarly, if you are unable to freely express emotions you probably have a blocked or unbalanced Throat Chakra.

THIRD EYE CHAKRA – Your Third Eye Chakra assists with good intuition and intellect. It governs the functioning of your nose, ears, left eye, and your lower brain. It also controls your autonomic nervous system. Your Third Eye Chakra also controls your hypothalamus and your pituitary gland. If this chakra is not functioning correctly then you can develop diseases of your sinuses, ears and hearing, eyes and sight, endocrine glands, lower brain, and your autonomic nervous system. When this chakra is out of balance you might find yourself making poor life choices because your judgment is clouded since you cannot see well.

By opening and balancing your Third Eye you are able to make a connection with your highest self, which will allow for the formation of reasonable and sound decisions. The elevated effectiveness of the sixth sense will give you the ability to gather information currently outside of your sensory range, the range usually considered to be abnormal for most people. A higher level of thought will enable the acquisition of desired goals and dreams by giving you the mental ability to fully see the bigger picture and knowing how to get it.

Having a better mental balance will lead to less fear of the unknown and will make it easier for you to get out of thoughts and situations negative by nature. By opening this chakra, you will gain real balance in your life and eliminate your unreasonable fears by trusting your intuition when it sends important messages regarding life events. A blocked or unbalanced Third Eye will make it seem like any action is insignificant, and it may cause you to struggle with depression and finding the greater purpose in your life.

When your Third Eye is healthy and balanced there is a greater ability to feel and have intuition, guidance, perception, awareness, and greater insight.

CROWN CHAKRA – Your Crown Chakra is found on the very top of your head, and it takes care of your right eye, your higher brain, and your pineal gland. It is in charge of emotions like self-realization and consciousness. When this chakra is not functioning correctly diseases of your cerebral cortex and your pineal gland can develop. When your Crown Chakra is not healthy you will feel boredom, alienation, or depression. You may feel confused in your life or be unable to concentrate. And when you are unable, or unwilling, to do the things you should be doing, you tend to close off your Crown Chakra, which causes a loss of connection with the rest of the chakras in your body including the higher powers in the universe. If this chakra is weak, you might start to create unreasonable phobias or create fear where none exists. It may be difficult to enjoy even the smallest pleasures in life.

Even minor disturbances in your chakras and your health will cause disturbances in your body that will appear as physical symptoms and manifestations. These symptoms will appear in your organs associated with that chakra. This does not mean the chakras are physical or physiological by nature, but rather your chakras are centers of energy exerting influence on you at many levels, including biological and physical levels. If even one of your centers of energy is off balance or unhealthy, you may see symptoms of disease or illnesses. Your chakras function much like a pendulum and if one chakra is not centered, the pendulum is thrown off its balance. This disturbance will be felt at the level of that chakra and even at the level of the chakras above and below the injured chakra.

Balancing and opening your Crown Chakra will give you the ability to connect with your consciousness in the universe and to experience that consciousness inside. True enlightenment will be gained as the truth of who you really are becomes known to you. A much greater overall connection to the universe and the world at large will be gained through this balancing process, and the knowledge of your universal consciousness will be open to you. Once your mind is open the physical world can be transcended and the realization that there is life beyond the physical world will be felt. The Crown Chakra is vital in achieving a sense of peace and comfort and in creating a life worth living and loving. It connects your whole being to the greater universe, using knowledge, bliss, acceptance, understanding, and information. Any imbalances or blockages in this chakra may reveal themselves as psychological problems.

Your chakras can be thrown off balance or made unhealthy by the rigors of daily life, but they are easily rebalanced and kept healthy with just a bit of attention. Their function can be regulated through the use of relaxation techniques, diet, exercise, meditation, and exercises in breathing. When your chakras are balanced by doing things physical in nature, then the function of the chakras is supported at many underlying levels. Rebalancing and keeping your chakras healthy supports your whole being physically, emotionally, psychologically, and spiritually. And by supporting your body the entire chakra system is supported, which in turn supports your entire body.

CONCLUSION

Thank you for making it through to the end of *Complete Chakras for Beginners:*
The Solution to Chakras Healing and Balancing Your Body, Mind, and Positive Energies. Let's hope it was informative and able to provide you with all of the tools you need to achieve your goals, whatever they may be.

The next step is to begin your journey into the world of the chakras and chakra healing. Take the things you learned in this book and use them to your advantage. You will be able to experience the kind of life you probably only dreamed about. You will find yourself happier and healthier than ever before. You will have the mental and physical energy to make it through each day and have energy left over. The chakras have a tremendous effect on the physical, mental, emotional, and spiritual parts of your being.

Note from the Author: Reviews are gold to authors! If you've enjoyed this book, would you consider rating it and reviewing it on Amazon?

If you would also like to be notified of more great releases, be privy to advance copy, and get great promotional discounts go here: https://completechakras.com   and drop me your details

For a limited time, I'm offering *Desmunde Dunne Yoga Made Easy* for free. This is a yoga classic and a must for those who want to learn yoga or learn to develop spiritually. A must for anybody's library!

Claim your free Yoga eBook: https://completechakras.com

REFERENCES

An Easy Beginners Guide to Chakra Meditation. (2019, January 25). Retrieved from https://blog.mindvalley.com/chakra-meditation/

Anna. (n.d.). Unicorn Crystals: 7 Gems Attuned to Their Realm. Retrieved from https://www.llewellyn.com/blog/2019/11/unicorn-crystals-7-gems-attuned-to-their-realm/

Chubé, A. (2015, March 23). Unicorns and Reiki. Retrieved from https://reikirays.com/19999/unicorns-and-reiki/

Crystals for Unicorn Energy. (n.d.). Retrieved from https://www.crystal-life.com/crystals-unicorn-energy/

Healing with the Unicorns. (n.d.). Retrieved from https://www.elementalbeings.co.uk/unicorns/healing-unicorns/

Kuna, A. (n.d.). Unicorns. Retrieved from http://www.nataliakuna.com/the-spiritual-energy-of-unicorns.html

ABOUT THE AUTHOR

Tracey is a natural intuitive Energy Healer and has been since a young age, and it's here where her passion lies. She studied energy systems for over 10 years, becoming qualified in Angelic Reiki and Reiki healing practices so she is able to utilize her skills for the benefit of others. She is an established Angelic Reiki Healer and energy worker, working with energy and chakras on a daily basis.

She is passionate about working with energy, calling it the "you energy," meaning chakra energy. Tracey firmly believes, that if used correctly– along with other modalities– it can be a game changer. She believes *using the body's own energy system can genuinely change lives on the physical, emotional and mental levels.*"

In addition to her energy healing she also had a long career in education, working closely with young people and adults to help them develop their abilities and skills. She also worked alongside small businesses, coaching and helping them develop and improve their skills. She is a qualified trainer and holds a Post Graduate Degree in Learning Development.

In the early years she practiced privately. But it wasn't until she teamed up with Anne Scholes that she became more open about her abilities. She met Anne on the show *Psychic Today*, where Anne is an established International Psychic Medium. Having much in common and both being healers, Anne and Tracey became great friends. Tracey now works independently and with Anne at her practice in the North of England. Tracey has years of experience in this area, offering individual intuitive healing sessions, teaching and consulting with groups. Offering these gifts helps clients and groups make real and positive change in their lives.

Her inspiration for this book comes from students and clients seeking advice and guidance on self-help techniques, drawing on her knowledge of energy and the chakra system, and how it all connects. The book is designed to be a simple way to connect the dots, while providing sign posting for other modalities, that may be beneficial.

The author can be contacted at:
completechakras@germon.co.uk

Printed in Poland
by Amazon Fulfillment
Poland Sp. z o.o., Wrocław

56742735R00092